ACUPRESSURE
FOR
ATHLETES

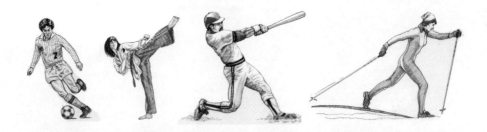

ACUPRESSURE

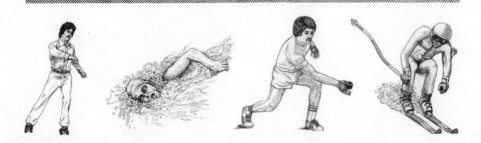

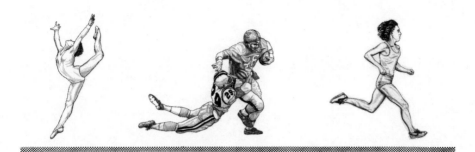

FOR ATHLETES

David J. Nickel

Foreword by Karlis C. Ullis, M.D.
Illustrated by Kira Od

An Owl Book
Henry Holt and Company   New York

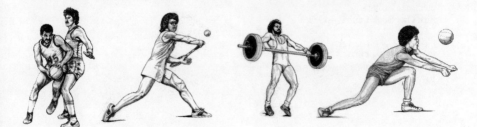

Published by Henry Holt and Company, Inc.,
115 West 18th Street, New York, New York 10011.
Published in Canada by Fitzhenry & Whiteside Limited,
195 Allstate Parkway, Markham, Ontario L3R 4T8.

Library of Congress Cataloging-in-Publication Data
Nickel, David J.
Acupressure for athletes.
Reprint. Originally published: Santa Monica, CA:
Health-Acu-Press, 1984.
"An Owl book."
Bibliography: p.
Includes index.
1. Acupressure.   2. Sports—Accidents and injuries—
Treatment.   3. Sports medicine.   I.   Title.
RM723.A27N53   1987   615.8′22   86-12097
ISBN 0-8050-0128-X (pbk.)

Henry Holt books are available at special discounts
for bulk purchases for sales promotions, premiums,
fund-raising, or educational use. Special editions
or book excerpts can also be created to specification.

    For details contact:

    Special Sales Director
    Henry Holt and Company, Inc.
    115 West 18th Street
    New York, New York 10011

First published by Health-Acu-Press in 1984; revised edition
published in 1985.
First Owl Book Edition—1987

Interior design: Lee Perry
Illustrator: Kira Od
Printed in the United States of America
10 9 8 7 6 5 4 3 2

To all athletes and sports enthusiasts,
to help you play better, feel stronger
and prevent injuries naturally.

Acknowledgments

I especially thank my mother, Agnes Nickel,
for her life-long inspiration, love and support.

Additionally I thank
for professional advice and assistance

Karlis Ullis, M.D.
Whitfield Reaves, O.M.D.
Elizabeth Austin, O.M.D.
Deke Kendall, O.M.D., Ph.D.
John Harris, M.T.
Nora Haber, R.N.
Debra Petersen, R.N.

for encouragement and support

Patricia Allen, Don Brosseau, Fa Cheng Chung,
Suk Wah Chung, Home Federal Savings, Winnie Lau,
Pak Wah Ng, Brian Nickel, Ruth Quenzer,
Steve and Sheryl Quenzer and Gordon Rose

**for professional knowledge
and guidance in the production of this book**

Gwendolyn Sze Chin Shim,
Nancy Allen, Patricia Bacall, Jack Booker,
Carolyn Goldsmith, Ellen Herbert, Linda McCrerey,
Joan Peters and Paul Whitehouse

Preface

Whether you are a weekend amateur or professional athlete, you run the risk of suffering one of the 17 million injuries per year in the United States that cost an estimated $40 billion in medical expenses. The skillful use of acupressure can free you from useless pain and high medical costs. It can help you relax, extend your limits and reach your performance goals. With acupressure, your finger can become a powerful tool to increase your abilities as an athlete.

The beauty of acupressure is that you can begin to use it immediately after an injury. It is a very safe self-help method, which cannot harm you or be overdone. It costs you nothing to use and can be done anywhere and anytime you choose.

For years I searched for a well-illustrated, easy-to-follow manual that would make acupressure available to athletes. Not finding one, I have written this book. The research has been a wonderful learning experience. Now I want to share the information with all who are interested in improving their health.

Even though the statistics on acupuncture are extensive, the studies on acupressure are really just beginning. I encourage athletes, trainers, coaches, physicians and scientists to explore, use and document the effectiveness of acupressure. The more information becomes available, the easier it will be to chart the success of acupressure in improving performance and treating injuries.

Have more fun playing—treat yourself!

David J. Nickel

DR. DAVID J. NICKEL
1987

Foreword

I am most happy to welcome Dr. David J. Nickel's book, *Acupressure for Athletes*, as a step forward in our continuing evolution toward self-regulation of human bodily functions. Now we have an easy-to-follow manual showing how to decrease pain, aid the healing process, speed recovery from training and prevent injury - thereby resulting in improved athletic performance. Acupressure treatments are simple, non-toxic, effective and have no harmful side effects. Dr. Nickel's book is the first of its kind to make such information available to the general public.

Fortunately, pressure point procedures are understood around the world, verified by voluminous scientific research over the last 15 years in the USA and Western Europe. The supporting scientific data and the physical, chemical and electrical basis of acupuncture are well established.

Having practiced sports medicine at UCLA since 1978, I have kept up with the latest scientific developments in this multi-disciplinary field. My personal study of acupuncture dates back to 1972, when I was a medical post graduate research fellow at the University of Washington School of Medicine. I have been a staff physician at numerous international sports events, one of the more memorable being the XXIII Summer Olympic Games in Los Angeles in 1984. Working with athletes in 23 different sports allowed me to observe and document acupressure and acupuncture to be effective for pain control, promotion of healing and more rapid recovery from training sessions.

The scientific community recognizes that acupuncture needling and electro-acutherapy are in some ways superior to acupressure. However, it is not feasible, practical or legal to perform these more technical medical practices, without extensive training. Therefore, *Acupressure for Athletes* becomes very important from a practical point of view for the recreational to professional athlete.

Because of its general application, *Acupressure for Athletes* represents a major breakthrough in our on-going pursuit of greater personal access to and control of our physiological functions. It is the first book to demonstrate the use of self-help acupressure for warm-up, cool-down, pre-competition and general body balancing. The use of Dr. Nickel's techniques allows for better utilization of the body's inherent self-regulating mechanism.

Acupressure for Athletes is an excellent, practical manual that can help trainers, coaches and all types of athletes reduce pain and promote physical harmony, thereby improving performance, naturally.

KARLIS ULLIS, MD
Assistant Clinical Professor
UCLA School of Medicine

UCLA Student Health Service
UCLA Medical Center
Los Angeles, California 90024

Medical Director
Sports Medicine Group
Pacific Palisades, California

1. Han, J.S. and L. Terenius. "Neuro-chemical Basis of Acupuncture Analgesia." *Annual Review of Pharmacological Toxology.* Vol. 22, 193-220, 1982.
2. Becker, Robert O. and Andrew A. Marino. *Electromagnetism and Life.* State University of New York Press, 1982.
3. Ulett, George A. *Principles and Practices of Physiologic Acupuncture.* Warren H. Green, Inc., 1982.
4. Pomeranz, Bruce and Daryl Chiu. "Naloxone Blockade of Acupuncture Analgesia: Endorphin Implicated." *Life Sciences,* 19 (11), 1976.
5. Looney, Gerald L. "A Neurologic Basis for Acupuncture." *Acupuncture and Electro-therapeutic Research: The International Journal.* I (1-4), 1975-6.

Table
of
Contents

Pain Chart

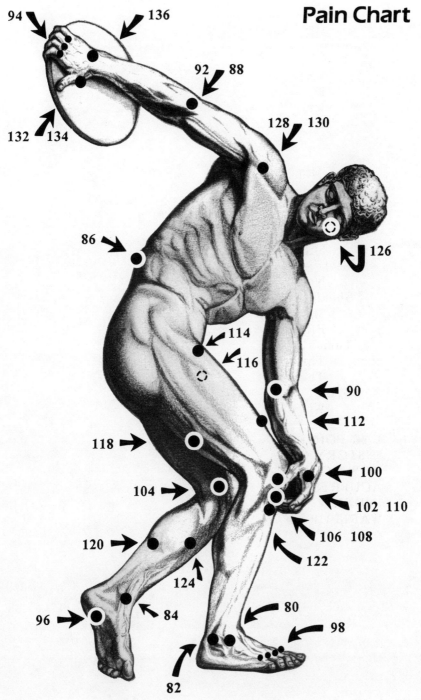

Introduction

You will find acupressure exciting and fun to explore. It has been available for thousands of years and is yours to use now. By creating a basic training program including acupressure for warm-up, cool-down, pre-competition stimulation and body balancing, which is supported by acupressure for injury prevention and treatment, you add to your competence and effectiveness as an athlete. By using your own hands, you carry with you always the tools to heal and the keys to health. Empower yourself to keep your body finely-tuned and injury-free. Treat yourself!

Maximizing Your Performance

Acupressure for Athletes provides you as an athlete — no matter what your ability level — with an amazing *new* tool that helps you to perform your sport at your personal maximum. This is accomplished by acupressure techniques for warm-up, pre-competition and body balancing.

Now you can design an *Acupressure Warm-Up* routine for your sports interests and your body's strengths and weaknesses. The warm-up includes your current stretching and warm-up procedures, along with acupressure techniques that enhance circulation, flexibility and muscle function and take only a few minutes of your time. By thoroughly warming-up, you can perform at your peak. You also take steps toward preventing injuries that keep you from getting out and having fun.

Stimulation of the *Pre-Competition* acupressure points can make a significant contribution toward your success by promoting the properly balanced physical, mental and psychological attitudes that are so frequently reported by winners. The stress of competition demands a well-trained and superbly conditioned body. In major competitions, however, the physical capabilities of the athletes are very close and the true challenge is the psychological one. Create your own *on* days!

1

Acupressure Body Balancing Points are given to help you alleviate many of the annoying conditions that limit your enjoyment, relaxation and performance during athletic activities. Sleep problems, menstrual discomfort, muscle tension and many other disturbances may be treated with acupressure techniques — by you.

Treating Your Injuries

Acupressure for Athletes also supports your right to understand and participate in your body's healing processes as actively as you engage in training and competition. Sprains and strains are the most common athletic injuries and can be quickly, safely and effectively treated with the step-by-step directions given in this text. Conventional first aid treatment is described in conjunction with the acupressure techniques in order to complete your knowledge of acceptable treatments. You also find clear explanations of what happens in your body when you sprain a ligament or strain a muscle or tendon. Understanding the healing processes within your body and the time they require allows you to be patient and not to stress your body too soon, thus possibly re-injuring yourself or aggravating a previous injury.

Athletes all over the world have an intense desire to perform to the best of their talent and training. Although this goal is most dramatically illustrated every four years in the competition at the Olympic Games, it is also seen in marathon runners, participants in the pick-up basketball game on Saturday afternoons, professional athletes in a world series or super bowl and every individual who exercises regularly for fun and fitness. As athletes, you are all looking for new ways to practice more effectively, improve your performance and above all to avoid injuries which prevent you from competing.

Comparing Acupressure and Massage

Among the *new* techniques for improving performance are two that have a long and respected history in the healing arts. Massage and acupressure have been known to reduce pain and swelling, improve circulation and speed healing of injuries. More athletes are realizing now, however, that these are also valuable methods of improving flexibility and performance. Many top-class athletes train only if they have regular massages. They attribute their ability to workout hard and to recuperate fast to the use of massage as a part of their training program.

Compared to acupressure, massage has three major drawbacks. First, it is not an appropriate immediate treatment for acute athletic injuries, such as sprains and strains. Over a recently injured area, it will usually increase pain and swelling and possibly cause other damage such as increased bleeding in the area of the injury. Second, it requires more time than acupressure. And third, to be most effective, it must be given by someone else. Acupressure is a precise way to deal with pain and swelling immediately, which does not put pressure directly on the injured area. It is also quick to perform and effectively done by yourself.

The ancient Chinese martial artists used their bodies vigorously, thus increasing their chance of injury. Over the centuries martial arts teachers developed a specific system of immediate first aid for their students by using hands and fingers to apply pressure to special points called *Judo Revival Points*. The Chinese discovered through experience that stimulation of certain points on the body has a defined and repeatable effect even on remote parts of the body — thus injuries can be treated without applying pressure to the injury itself. This is acupressure.

For athletic injuries such as sprains and strains, acupressure overcomes the difficulties encountered in using massage. Acupressure is a technique that can be confidently employed at any time, even immediately after an injury has occurred. With precise use of acupressure you have a safe, reliable option that can help you take an active part in healing yourself if you suffer an injury.

In his editorial *The Neglected Art of Massage,* Allan J. Ryan, MD and Editor-in-Chief of *The Physician and Sportsmedicine,* states that, "Massage before exercise apparently improves muscular performance." And that, "massage following exercise is restorative in that it promotes a state of general relaxation. It reduces muscle tension, relieves swelling and helps prevent soreness."

And yet, Dr. Ryan regrets that even though massage does improve muscular performance, "today most (athletes) will never receive one (massage) unless they are recovering from an injury. The basic forms of massage are familiar to trainers and physical therapists, yet the technique is seldom used. Massage has been neglected principally because of time limitations, not because it is ineffective. Most trainers must provide a variety of services for dozens, even hundreds, of athletes. A good massage may take 15 to 30 minutes, depending on the purpose.

An effective *Acupressure Warm-Up* or *Cool-Down* may take as little as 5 minutes. And best of all, you do it yourself!

Succeeding with Acupressure

Eleven world records were set at the International Powerlifting Championships in Hawaii on March 3, 1985. Nine of which were preceded with acupressure pre-competition treatments. Ed Coan broke 5 world records that day. He requested treatments for muscle tightness and cramping. After having him drink a little warm water before each event, I treated the following points: *Fighting Spirit* (p 50), *Go Power* (p 51), and *Competitive Edge* (p 51). Ed later told reporters on camera, "I want to especially thank Dr. Nickel and his acupressure treatments — that helped me break these world records today."

Here's another personal experience from the Masters Swimming Championships, Industry Hills, California, May 26-28, 1984. I gave pre-competition acupressure and acupuncture treatments to 68 swimmers who reported on their results. Based on a total of 56 acupressure treatments, 35 (or 62.5%) resulted in best-ever times and 4 (or 7.5%) resulted in ties of best previous times. No one reported performing worse following pre-competition treatment. Those who previously had pain were amazed that they could compete pain-free following the acupressure.

A 72 year old master swimmer, at the same competition, had so much back pain after her first race, that she decided not to compete in the other events for which she was scheduled. At that

4

point she heard that I was giving ear acupressure treatments and came to see me. After treatment, her muscles felt stronger. She decided to compete in her last relay event. She did so with no pain and with one of her best times ever. "It's amazing! Why didn't I come to you sooner? I could have competed in all my events!"

During my coaching days at Palmdale High School, my best gymnast was just about to complete her final floor exercise, when she said, "Coach, I don't want to compete. I'm tired; I feel lousy; and I know I will do terrible." I did a quick 10 second pre-competition stimulation treatment, using the *Fighting Spirit Point* (p 50). She felt better immediately and won first place.

At the '84 Summer Games at Mt. SAC, San Antonio College, Walnut, California, I treated a Canadian 100 meter Olympic hurdler. He had no specific health or injury complaints, but his left gluteus maximus muscle tested weak before ear acupressure and strong afterwards. Only 45 minutes later, he did his best hurdle time ever!

Weight and/or appetite control are frequently important issues for athletes. I have treated hundreds of weekend athletes by having them stimulate the appetite center in the brain via a point in their ear, the *Hunger Point* (p 56). Most wished to lose weight and reported feeling easily in control of their appetite, a reduction of appetite and/or feeling full from eating less than usual. For those wanting to gain weight, the same point can be used since the stimulation of the brain has a balancing effect.

Recent magazine articles document the effectiveness of acupressure in treating conditions of concern to athletes. In the March 1981 *The Physician and Sportsmedicine,* an article entitled *Acupressure Massage to Relieve Menstrual Cramps* explains how to keep female athletes in active training and competition without monthly discomfort.

In the *Sportsmedicine Book*, Gabe Mirkin and Marshall Hoffman give exact directions for treating stitches in the side, which use acupressure without calling it by name. "What should you do when you get a stitch? Slow down and push your fingers deep into the site of the pain, usually just below the last rib on the right upper part of your belly. Bend forward and exhale, pursing your lips.

The pain will disappear soon and you can continue running."

A recent example of the use of acupressure to heal athletic injuries was mentioned by Kerry Lynch, a United States Nordic combined skier in the 1984 Winter Olympics in Sarajevo. During a television interview he gave credit to his acupressurist for aiding in the rehabilitation of his knee which allowed him to successfully compete in the Olympics.

Acupressure has a wide range of medical uses. Modern Chinese doctors have performed thousands of medical operations, such as tooth extractions, tonsillectomies, thyroid surgeries and stomach surgeries, utilizing acupressure as the sole or primary method of anesthesia. In 90% of the cases, there is little to no pain! (See *First Medical College of PLA*, p 154.)

The safe and simple act of applying pressure to certain parts of the body can provide results that may substitute for many medical prescription and non-prescription drugs which seem effective but may have undesirable side-effects. Drug therapy generally shuts off and inhibits that aspect of the body's immune system for which it substitutes, whereas acupressure turns on the body's immuno-defense system. Narcotic medications shut down the production of the body's hormones; yet acupressure stimulates the body to supply its own needed pain-killing chemicals. Narcotics are addictive. The body's own *high* is natural and healthy!

Acupressure is not the only way to stimulate your brain hormones and experience a natural *high* — acupuncture, vigorous physical exercise, massage, laughter, sex and meditation can also create some of the same beneficial and desirable responses. (See *How Acupressure Works,* pp 143 to 148.)

The above successes emphasize that acupressure is an option any athlete can use as part of an over-all health maintenance and training program. Acupressure is the preferred, quick, safe and simple self-help technique to maximize performance and treat sprains and strains.

Acupressure Technique

We all instinctively touch, rub or press on a sore muscle or injured body part to relieve pain. Healers in many ancient countries, including China, Egypt, Greece and India, discovered that stimulation or pressure on certain points of the body often produces a reduction of pain and swelling, and thus shortens healing time. They also made the amazing discovery that stimulating particular points effects other, remote parts of the body!

The technique of acupressure involves applying pressure with the thumb or finger tips to specific points on the body, in order to reduce pain, to improve circulation, flexibility and muscle function and to promote body balance and healing.

The pressure can be applied to the surface of the disturbed area, to the corresponding left/right body part and/or to a remote but related point. The hands and ears contain many points that effect distant body parts and are easily accessible. Therefore, many acupressure treatments may be directed solely to these areas and efficiently treat any part of the body. The mannner in which the pressure is applied can help determine whether the effect is one of stimulation (short duration and/or pinching pressure) or relaxation (longer duration and/or steady pressure). Also certain of the points by their nature, seem to be more stimulating or relaxing.

An acupressure treatment can be given immediately after an injury and can be effective for an indefinite period of time, depending on the general health of the individual and the amount of stress placed on the body. There is no need to produce additional pain or internal bleeding by applying acupressure directly to an acute injury, as a corresponding body part or remote point can be even more effective for treatment than the actual site of the injury.

Treatment can be performed by anyone with a knowledge of the appropriate acupressure points, because there is no risk of injury due to stimulating a wrong point, only lessened effectiveness. Acupressure can produce results quickly and is easy to learn. Treatment on one's self is easy to perform, unless an injury prevents this. In such cases, a friend can follow your directions and be your hands for you. It is usually easier to relax totally while someone else applies the acupressure.

Preparing and Relaxing

The degree to which you are relaxed will help determine the effectiveness of acupressure. Therefore, try to find a comfortable and quiet place to treat yourself. You may sit or lie down, whichever you find most convenient and relaxing. Deep breathing is a useful technique to help you become more relaxed. It is especially calming to breathe in through your nose and to forcefully exhale through your mouth. Visualizing strength and flexibility increasing and the pain of an injury decreasing and leaving your body promotes the beneficial results of acupressure.

During acupressure it is not necessary to remove any clothing. Loosening tight clothing, such as ties, belts, etc., increases circulation and enhances results. It is preferable for your hands to be clean and your fingernails trimmed. If your hands feel cold rub them together until they begin to feel warmer. For treatment of an injury, acupressure may be applied any time after you have begun to follow the general first aid procedures.

Applying Proper Pressure

Pressure can be applied with either the index finger or thumb. Sufficient pressure is usually more easily applied to the hand points with the thumb and to the ear points with the index finger. For body acupressure, use finger or thumb, whichever is most convenient or comfortable; a knuckle can be used to achieve greater pressure.

This book recommends two methods of applying pressure. For *Cool-Down, Body Balancing* and *Treatment*, the pressure should be applied slowly with a gradually increasing force. Apply the

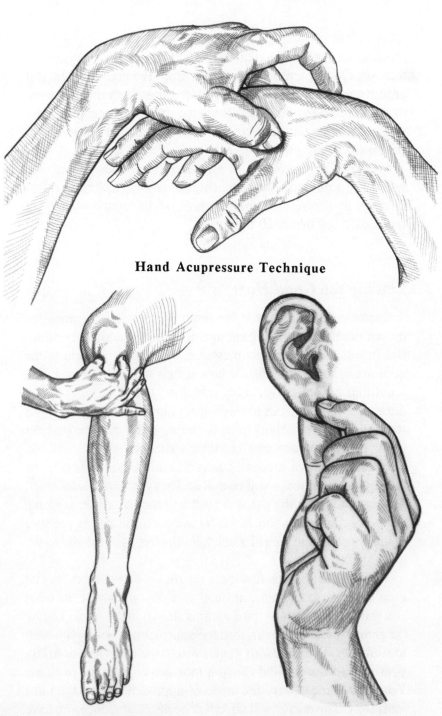

Hand Acupressure Technique

Body Acupressure Technique

Ear Acupressure Technique

pressure for 5 seconds and then gradually release the pressure for 5 seconds. Do not remove your finger from the point. Repeat this procedure usually for a total of 1 minute. Counting "one-ten thousand, two-ten thousand, three-ten thousand," etc. may help you determine the correct intervals. During an *Acupressure Warm-Up*, apply pressure to each point for 30 seconds.

For *Pre-Competition* — or any time stimulation rather than relaxation is desired — use a pinching or jabbing technique rather than steady pressure. Simply pinch or jab the acupressure point repeatedly and firmly 10 times.

Finding the *Good Hurt*

Successful acupressure is the result of accurately locating the proper point and applying enough pressure to adequately stimulate it. For an amateur acupressurist the only sure guide to the accurate location of a point is how it feels when stimulated. The sensations have been variously described as dull, aching, sore, a distended feeling, an electric feeling, numbness, burning, a hot and stinging feeling, etc. Many times the term *good hurt* is used to refer to the presence of any or all of these sensations.

In general, when pressing points on your hands and body the feeling you experience will be dull and achy in nature. However, pressing points in the ear will tend to produce a hot, stinging, almost burning sensation. Begin by using a firm rotating pressure in the approximate area of a point, let the feelings lead you to the exact point.

To locate ear points, first use a mirror — two mirrors may be even easier — to examine the outer area of your ear. Relate what you see in the mirror to the diagrams shown in the book. Locate the general areas of the ear, then the approximate points you wish to stimulate. The *good hurt* guides you to the exact location. Use your index finger to find the spot most sensitive to the pressure. You may want to vary the angle of approach to find the most sensitivity. The mirror will no longer be necessary, once you have succeeded in locating the proper point.

Be sure to press the points with sufficient firmness. The *good hurt* sensations can guide you in the proper pressure as well as location. You do not want to push so hard that you experience continuous pain or severe discomfort. If your skin starts to turn red, avoid possible bruising by moving on to another point. The skin turning red is another good sign that you have stimulated a point sufficiently. On ear points, you may use your fingernail, but be careful not to scratch or break the skin on your ear. Putting your thumb behind the ear while massaging is often helpful. On all points, the finger should not slide over the skin but instead keep firm contact and move the skin. If you feel you have not successfully located a point, re-check the illustration for the correct location. Then try more pressure.

Breathing in Time

When timing the pressure, 5 seconds on — 5 seconds off, synchronize your breathing so that you are exhaling through your mouth as you apply pressure. Inhale through your nose as you ease pressure. This should assure that your breathing is rhythmic, deep and relaxed. If the acupressure point you are stimulating is particularly sensitive and/or you are treating for a painful injury, it will be helpful to exhale forcefully as you push. Visualization plays an important part here. Visualize that you are blowing the pain away with each press.

Making the Most of Acupressure

During an acupressure treatment for injury, let the pain of the injury be your guide. You may stop the treatment at any time that you feel a significant reduction in the pain. Complete the full treatment if the pain keeps up, in fact you may even repeat certain steps or the whole treatment. *Never continue to follow a procedure that causes persistent pain in the area of your injury.*

After obtaining relief by using hand, ear or body acupressure, pain and aches may return temporarily after a period of time. This is a natural occurrence as part of the healing process.

As with any other medical procedure, there are certain situations when acupressure may not be suitable for you. If you have a heart problem be sure that you sit or lie down during the treatment as acupressure may at times make you feel faint. If you are pregnant consult a certified acupuncturist before using acupressure, because stimulation of certain points can cause uterine contractions. *Avoid using acupressure on bruises, scars, the eyeballs or any injured portion of the body.*

Several factors can minimize the results obtained from an acupressure treatment. If you have just eaten, better results may be obtained by waiting for an hour. But if you have not eaten for 5 to 6 hours, you may need to eat and then wait for an hour before beginning your treatment. You may find that being over-tired interferes with your ability to effectively benefit from acupressure.

And finally, since it can take years of training and practice to do acupressure expertly, do not hesitate to consult a licensed practitioner for advice and do not become discouraged if your initial attempts do not bring the results you hoped. You cannot cause harm by using incorrect acupressure points. The fact that you are willing to take your health in your own hands can only be a benefit. Once you gain experience with acupressure you will enjoy using this simple, safe and effective treatment and prevention technique.

The function of acupressure is to aid and encourage the body to correct its own imbalances. Therefore, it is most helpful in conjunction with a sensible fitness program that includes a nutritious diet, ample exercise and rest, and positive attitudes.

Maintaining Health

As an over-all program to maintain health, to help prevent and to help heal the tearing of ligament, muscle and tendon fibers, you may:

1. Stretch and warm-up adequately prior to physical activity and cool-down afterwards.
2. Use acupressure on a daily basis to strengthen injury-prone body parts or previously injured body parts.

3. Use acupressure as a warm-up before and a cool-down after physical activities to regulate circulation and improve muscle function.
4. Include aerobic exercise in your training program such as race-walking, jogging, dancing, swimming, biking, jumping-rope, re-bounding and strenuous yoga postures.
5. Increase training time and difficulty progressively.
6. Be careful not to over-train.
7. Keep muscles warm.
8. To prevent re-injury, allow time for healing of torn fibers and injured tissue before resuming strenuous athletics.
9. If possible after any sprain or strain, have a muscle test, i.e. applied kinesiology, prior to resuming strenuous physical activity.
10. For health maintenance eat a diet of cooked foods: primarily vegetables with some grains, meat, herbs and natural sweets. During the healing process emphasize foods that improve blood circulation, remove coagulation and enhance tissue repair. Vegetables: beets, corn, potatoes, leeks, eggplant, capers, kidney beans, chestnuts and pine nuts. Grains: rice (brown or long-grain white), oats and pearl barley. Meats: chicken, beef, liver, lamb kidney, tuna and sardines. Fruits: strawberries and figs. Herbs: white pepper, spearmint, rosemary, dill seed, bay leaf and marjoram. Sweets: molasses, malt sugar and rice bran syrup. During healing it is especially important to avoid foods and liquids that tend to cause blood congestion and reduce circulation. These include raw foods, such as fruits, juices and salads, also chilled and iced foods and liquids. Excessively spicy food, most nuts, chocolate, beer, citrus, white sugar, coffee, over-the-counter drugs, additives and preservatives increase stress on the nervous system and tend to slow healing.
11. Drink a cup/glass of warm water as soon as possible after an injury. Drink only warm to room-temperature liquids while in pain. Drink enough water to urinate 3 to 4 times per day.
12. Use natural agents like aloe vera, tiger balm, white flower oil and medical plasters two days after injury to increase circulation and movement of fluids from injury site.
13. Relax and enjoy learning what makes your body function best.

1

ACUPRESSURE FOR MAXIMIZING PERFORMANCE

Acupressure
Warm-Up
and Cool-Down

As an athlete you are vitally interested in maintaining fitness and preventing injury to your body. One of the best methods for achieving these goals is a thorough warm-up — one that insures your body has developed adequate circulation before meeting the demands of rigorous physical activity and competition.

An acupressure warm-up is a beneficial addition to your regular warm-up and stretching activities. A few minutes of time spent on the acupressure warm-up, just prior to your regular warm-up and stretching routine, rewards you with increased circulation, as well as improved flexibility and muscle function, and is your best safeguard against sprains and strains. You can use the acupressure points in this warm-up section both to stimulate your system before physical activity and to relax it after your workout.

Minimizing Your Warm-Up

A warm-up routine should be as individual as the athlete performing it. If you prefer a very brief acupressure warm-up, use the over-all warm-up points (p 21). These are the hand and body points that increase circulation, enhance brain-nerve-muscle communication and improve over-all body function. Follow this quick acupressure warm-up with your regular warm-up routine, which should take less time than usual. Then you're on your way!

Planning Your Personal Acupressure Warm-Up

Design a personal warm-up program for each sport in which you engage. Every sport stresses your body. And for each athletic activity, a certain type of injury is most common — usually sprains and strains. Also, certain body parts are most commonly injured. When you plan your *personal acupressure warm-up*, several questions should be answered. "What joints and muscles are stressed by the sport I am about to undertake?" "What parts of my body are most susceptible to injury from this sport?" "Have previous injuries left parts of my body at risk of re-injury?"

Turn to the pages for your chosen sport, they give you all the information you need to thoroughly familiarize yourself with which body parts are most stressed and most frequently injured during that sport. The injury information is taken from the *Consumer Product Safety Commission Hazard Identification and Analysis*, 1982. All traumatic injuries that require at least emergency room attention are reflected in this report. The number of actual injuries is estimated at three times the number of injuries reported by emergency rooms. The *Participants* figures are estimated totals taken from the 1982 *Sports Participation Study*, by the A.C. Nielson Company (except as otherwise noted).

Many sport injuries occur through over-use, rather than from accident or trauma. Examples are *Tennis Elbow, Pitcher's Elbow* and shoulder strain from swimming. These injuries are often not reported in the injury statistics. However, warm-up points for these body parts are included on the hand acupressure diagram. Follow the numbered sequence on the diagram to assure that you adequately warm-up.

Using the Warm-Up and Cool-Down Form

Tear out a blank *Warm-Up and Cool-Down Form* from the back of the book. (If you are involved in many sports and will be making several warm-up routines, photocopy the form before marking on it.)

Part 1 of the warm-up includes hand acupressure for at least the 3 body parts most frequently stressed by your sport. The acupressure points for these body parts are shown in the hand diagram for your sport. Circle and number the points on your *Warm-Up Form* to correspond with the points on the hand diagram.

17

Part 2 of your personal warm-up involves body acupressure. For your sport the body part that receives the most stress deserves extra attention. At the end of the hand acupressure warm-up instructions, for each sport, you are referred to the *Prevention* page in the *Acupressure Treatment* section where you are shown the proper body point/s to stimulate. Circle this point on the body diagram of your *Warm-Up Form* and place a number *1* by it.

If you have previous injuries that effect your performance, in a particular sport, the body part/s involved also deserve body acupressure during your warm-up for that sport. List the body part/s in Part 2 of the form and refer again to the *Treating Sprains and Strains* section for these specific injuries. Mark the points on the body diagram of your warm-up form. Number them in order of their importance, beginning with number *2*.

With this information on the form, you have created the basis for an *acupressure personal warm-up* designed for your body and a particular sport. It includes (1) hand acupressure for the 3 body parts most stressed, followed by (2) body acupressure for the most stressed body part.

An *expanded personal warm-up* could include all the hand points from the sport warm-up page and the body points for the most stressed body part and for your personal injuries. Additionally you may include the over-all warm-up points: *Muscle Flexibility, Ligament-Tendon Flexibility, Muscle Relaxing* and *Ligament-Tendon Relaxing* (p 21). Two of these are hand acupressure and two are body acupressure. To meet your individual needs and schedule, expand or shorten your warm-up as much as you wish.

Warming-Up

During Part 1 of your *personal acupressure warm-up*, use hand acupressure on points 1, 2, and 3 of the hand diagram. For Part 2, use body acupressure on the number 1 circled point. This takes approximately 5 minutes to perform.

For an *expanded personal warm-up*, first use all the circled hand points in order. Next, use all the body points in order. Also you may want to use the 4 over-all warm-up points.

18

Cooling-Down

After athletic activity, help your body more quickly adjust to a relaxed state with an acupressure cool-down. This is the most efficient way to return your body to its resting state and prepare it for further competition. For maximum results use the same points for cool-down as you do for a personal warm-up.

Or for a quick cool-down routine use the wrist and ear acupressure points: *Stage Fright* and *Muscle Relaxing* (p 47). These points are also beneficial when you feel pre-competition jitters. In fact, you can press these cool-down points any time you feel anxious, nervous or fearful.

NOTE: Acupressure warm-up and cool-down are not meant to replace your usual stretching, warming-up and cooling-down routines. Use the acupressure warm-up just prior to or with your regular warm-up procedures to enhance circulation, flexibility and readiness to perform. Similarly, use the acupressure cool-down points to begin your usual cooling-down routine. For the *Pre-Competition Acupressure Routine*, see pp 48 to 51.

WARM-UP ACUPRESSURE TECHNIQUE:

1. Apply continuous firm pressure to each warm-up point for 30 seconds: 5 seconds on - 5 seconds off. Begin with left side and repeat on the right side.
   - Move corresponding body part as pressure is applied, as appropriate.
   - Visualize the body becoming stronger and more flexible, while exhaling forcefully.
   - Relax your breathing.
2. Expect to feel:
   - Good hurt at the acupressure point.
   - Greater strength and flexibility.

COOL-DOWN ACUPRESSURE TECHNIQUE:

1. Apply continuous firm pressure to each ear point for 1 minute: 5 seconds on - 5 seconds off.
   - Begin with the left side, then repeat on the right side.
   - Visualize the body becoming more calm and the muscles becoming more relaxed and loose, while exhaling forcefully.
2. Expect to feel:
   - Good hurt at the acupressure point.
   - Greater calmness and the release of muscle tension.
3. If body does not feel significantly relaxed:
   - Repeat the procedure.
   - Have a friend hold firm pressue on the points.

20

OVER-ALL WARM-UP

Hand Acupressure

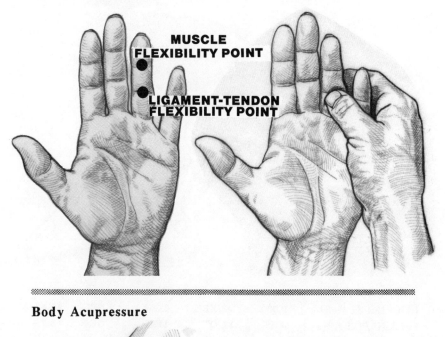

MUSCLE FLEXIBILITY POINT

LIGAMENT-TENDON FLEXIBILITY POINT

Body Acupressure

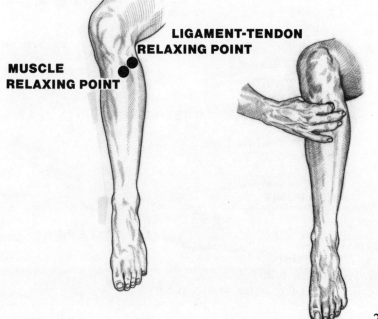

LIGAMENT-TENDON RELAXING POINT

MUSCLE RELAXING POINT

21

BADMINTON

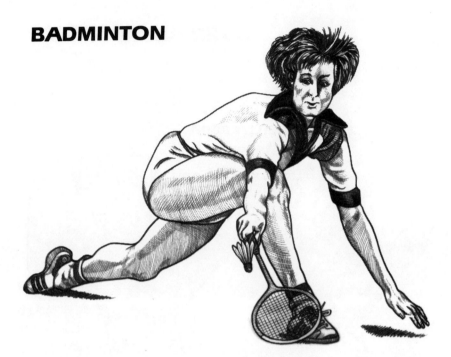

PARTICIPANTS	11,408	AREAS INJURED		CALF	11.9%
INJURIES	9,000	ANKLE	23.9%	KNEE	10.4%
SPRAINS/STRAINS	58.1%	FOOT	12.4%	TOE	8.5%

National Federation Handbook 83-84

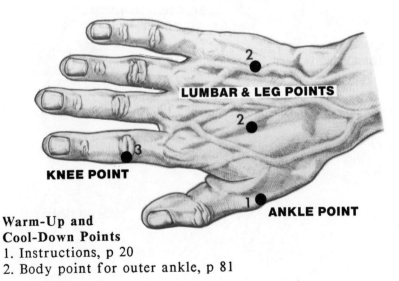

LUMBAR & LEG POINTS

KNEE POINT

ANKLE POINT

Warm-Up and
Cool-Down Points
1. Instructions, p 20
2. Body point for outer ankle, p 81

22

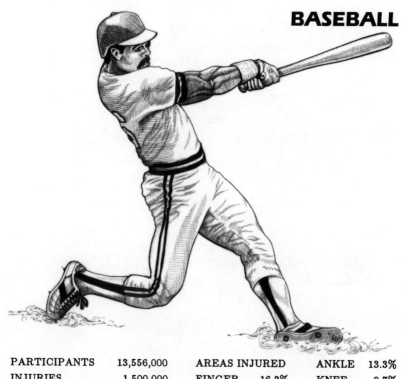

BASEBALL

PARTICIPANTS	13,556,000	AREAS INJURED		ANKLE	13.3%
INJURIES	1,500,000	FINGER	16.2%	KNEE	8.7%
SPRAINS/STRAINS	27.8%	FACE	13.8%	HEAD	5.4%

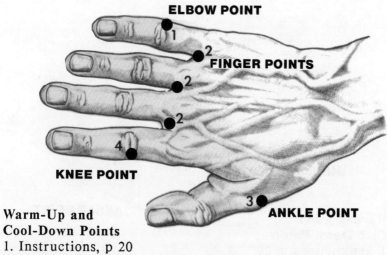

ELBOW POINT

FINGER POINTS

KNEE POINT

ANKLE POINT

**Warm-Up and
Cool-Down Points**
1. Instructions, p 20
2. Body point for inner elbow, p 91

23

BASKETBALL

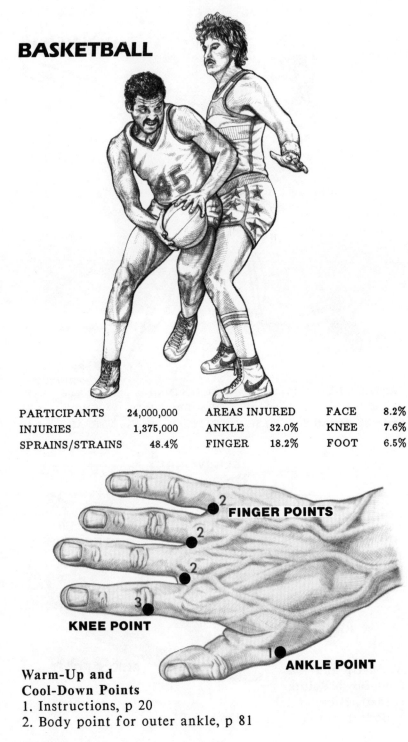

PARTICIPANTS	24,000,000	AREAS INJURED		FACE	8.2%
INJURIES	1,375,000	ANKLE	32.0%	KNEE	7.6%
SPRAINS/STRAINS	48.4%	FINGER	18.2%	FOOT	6.5%

FINGER POINTS

KNEE POINT

ANKLE POINT

Warm-Up and
Cool-Down Points
1. Instructions, p 20
2. Body point for outer ankle, p 81

BOWLING

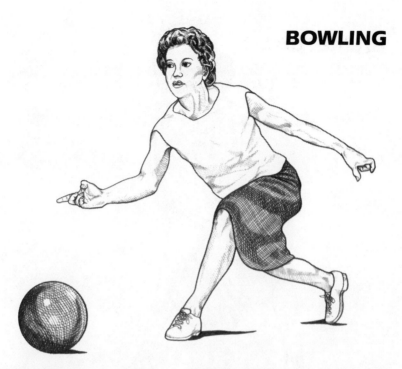

PARTICIPANTS	40,260,000	AREAS INJURED		L. TRUNK	9.7%
INJURIES	60,000	FINGER	23.4%	KNEE	9.3%
SPRAINS/STRAINS	48.4%	ANKLE	11.8%	WRIST	7.7%

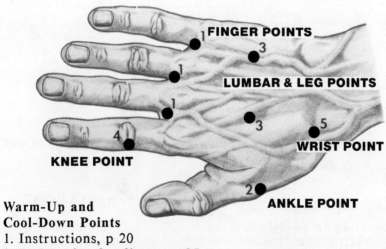

FINGER POINTS

LUMBAR & LEG POINTS

WRIST POINT

KNEE POINT

ANKLE POINT

Warm-Up and
Cool-Down Points
1. Instructions, p 20
2. Body point for finger, p 95

25

DANCE

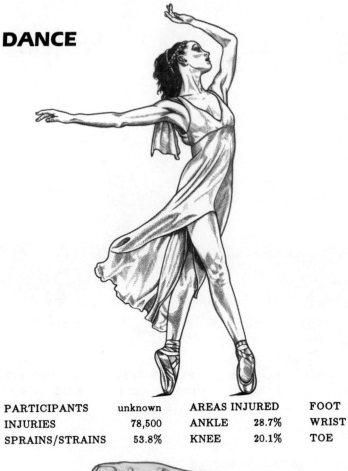

PARTICIPANTS	unknown	AREAS INJURED		FOOT	11.2%
INJURIES	78,500	ANKLE	28.7%	WRIST	5.6%
SPRAINS/STRAINS	53.8%	KNEE	20.1%	TOE	5.2%

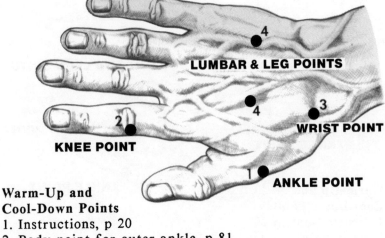

LUMBAR & LEG POINTS

WRIST POINT

KNEE POINT

ANKLE POINT

Warm-Up and
Cool-Down Points
1. Instructions, p 20
2. Body point for outer ankle, p 81

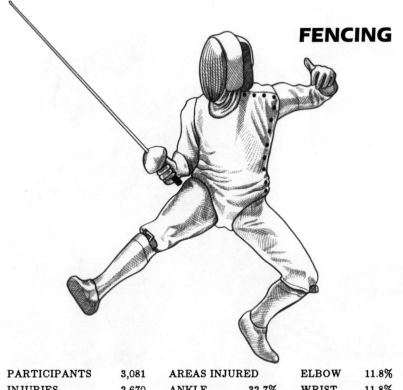

FENCING

PARTICIPANTS	3,081	AREAS INJURED		ELBOW	11.8%
INJURIES	2,670	ANKLE	32.7%	WRIST	11.8%
SPRAINS/STRAINS	26.7%	U. TRUNK	11.8%	FACE	11.8%

National Federation Handbook 83-84 and
National Collegiate Athletic Association 82-83

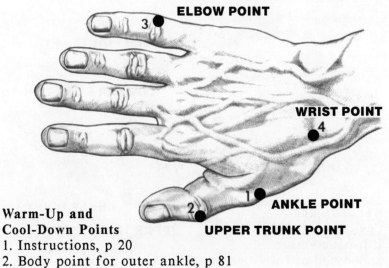

ELBOW POINT

WRIST POINT

ANKLE POINT

UPPER TRUNK POINT

Warm-Up and
Cool-Down Points
1. Instructions, p 20
2. Body point for outer ankle, p 81

FOOTBALL

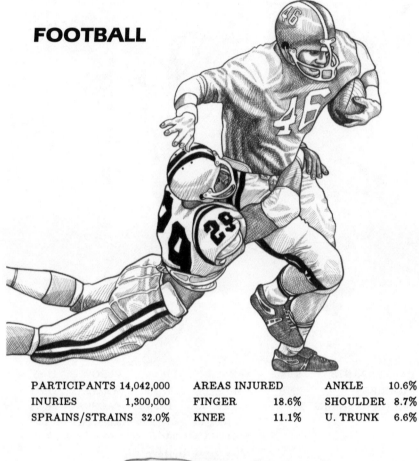

PARTICIPANTS 14,042,000	AREAS INJURED		ANKLE	10.6%
INURIES 1,300,000	FINGER	18.6%	SHOULDER	8.7%
SPRAINS/STRAINS 32.0%	KNEE	11.1%	U. TRUNK	6.6%

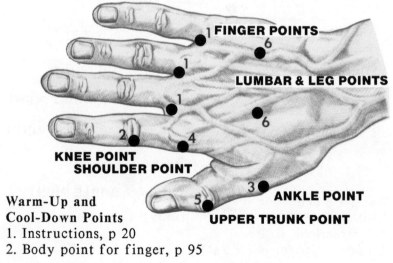

FINGER POINTS

LUMBAR & LEG POINTS

KNEE POINT
SHOULDER POINT

ANKLE POINT

UPPER TRUNK POINT

Warm-Up and
Cool-Down Points
1. Instructions, p 20
2. Body point for finger, p 95

28

GOLF

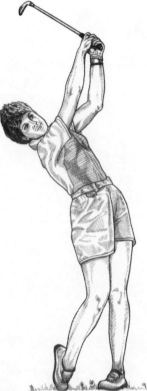

PARTICIPANTS	17,367,000	AREAS INJURED		ANKLE	9.4%
INJURIES	63,000	FACE	25.0%	WRIST	6.5%
SPRAINS/STRAINS	20.3%	HEAD	18.7%	MOUTH	5.5%

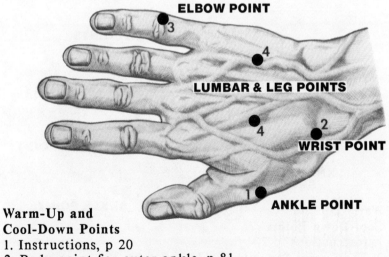

ELBOW POINT

3

4

LUMBAR & LEG POINTS

4   2

WRIST POINT

1

ANKLE POINT

**Warm-Up and
Cool-Down Points**
1. Instructions, p 20
2. Body point for outer ankle, p 81

GYMNASTICS

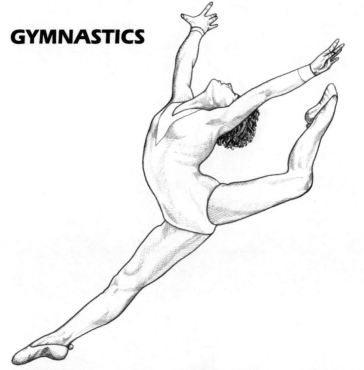

PARTICIPANTS	unknown	AREAS INJURED		FINGER	9.3%
INJURIES	160,000	ANKLE	12.7%	FOOT	8.7%
SPRAINS/STRAINS	40.9%	WRIST	11.1%	L. TRUNK	5.4%

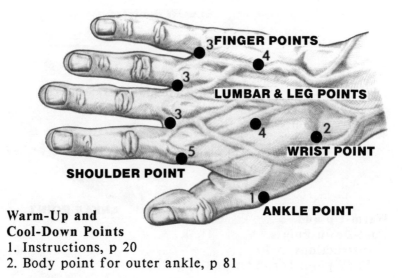

Warm-Up and Cool-Down Points
1. Instructions, p 20
2. Body point for outer ankle, p 81

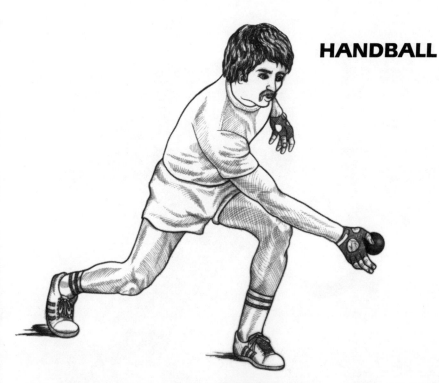

HANDBALL

PARTICIPANTS	2,634,000	AREAS INJURED		HAND	9.5%
INJURIES	12,000	ANKLE	29.2%	FACE	9.4%
SPRAINS/STRAINS	39.7%	FINGER	11.2%	KNEE	7.8%

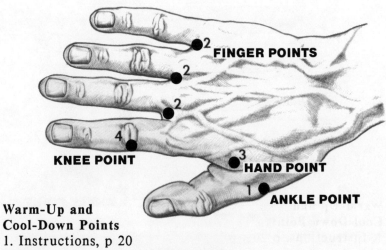

FINGER POINTS

KNEE POINT

HAND POINT

ANKLE POINT

**Warm-Up and
Cool-Down Points**
1. Instructions, p 20
2. Body point for outer ankle, p 81

ICE HOCKEY

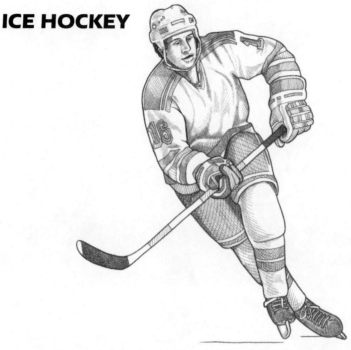

PARTICIPANTS	1,381,000	AREAS INJURED		SHOULDER	7.1%
INJURIES	68,997	FACE	29.6%	ANKLE	6.5%
SPRAINS/STRAINS	28.9%	KNEE	9.5%	MOUTH	6.3%

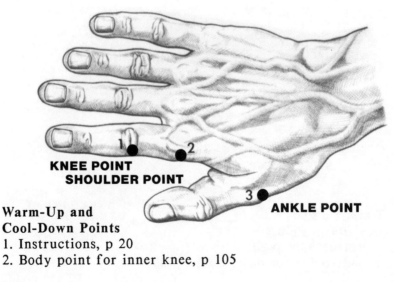

KNEE POINT
SHOULDER POINT
ANKLE POINT

**Warm-Up and
Cool-Down Points**
1. Instructions, p 20
2. Body point for inner knee, p 105

MARTIAL ARTS

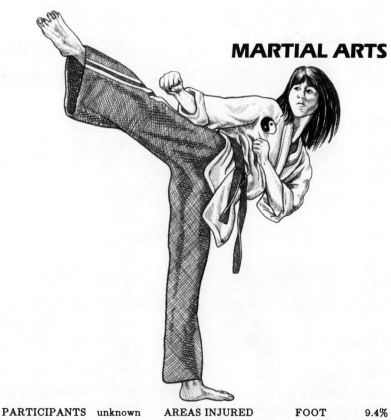

PARTICIPANTS	unknown	AREAS INJURED		FOOT	9.4%
INJURIES	62,000	FACE	11.7%	SHOULDER	8.8%
SPRAINS/STRAINS	22.9%	FINGER	10.6%	U. TRUNK	7.3%

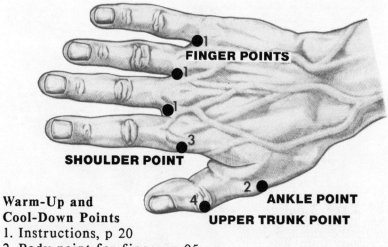

FINGER POINTS

SHOULDER POINT

ANKLE POINT

UPPER TRUNK POINT

Warm-Up and Cool-Down Points
1. Instructions, p 20
2. Body point for finger, p 95

33

RACQUETBALL

PADDLEBALL

SQUASH

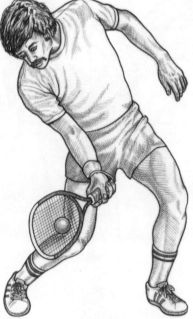

PARTICIPANTS	12,456,000	AREAS INJURED		EYEBALL	6.4%
INJURIES	106,000	FACE	22.3%	FOOT	6.3%
SPRAINS/STRAINS	38.0%	ANKLE	20.6%	KNEE	3.7%

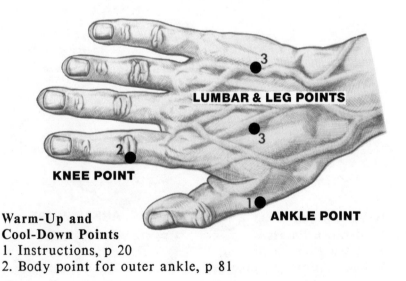

LUMBAR & LEG POINTS

KNEE POINT

ANKLE POINT

Warm-Up and
Cool-Down Points
1. Instructions, p 20
2. Body point for outer ankle, p 81

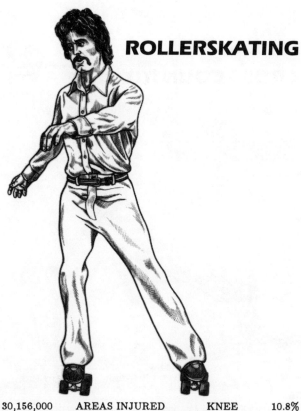

ROLLERSKATING

PARTICIPANTS	30,156,000	AREAS INJURED		KNEE	10.8%
INJURIES	438,000	WRIST	24.8%	ELBOW	9.8%
SPRAINS/STRAINS	25.5%	FOREARM	10.8%	ANKLE	7.6%

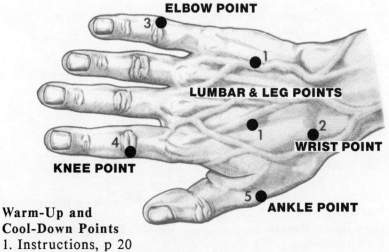

ELBOW POINT

LUMBAR & LEG POINTS

WRIST POINT

KNEE POINT

ANKLE POINT

Warm-Up and
Cool-Down Points
1. Instructions, p 20
2. Body point for back, p 87

SKIING:
CROSS-COUNTRY

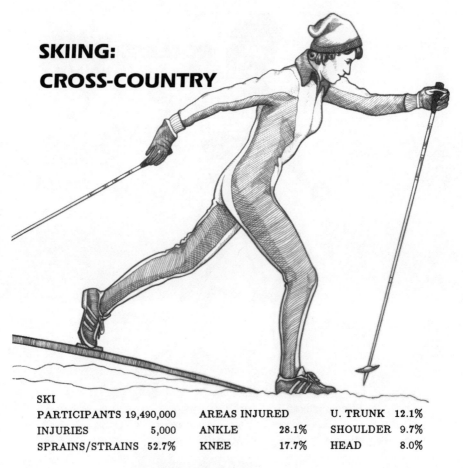

SKI

		AREAS INJURED		U. TRUNK	12.1%
PARTICIPANTS	19,490,000				
INJURIES	5,000	ANKLE	28.1%	SHOULDER	9.7%
SPRAINS/STRAINS	52.7%	KNEE	17.7%	HEAD	8.0%

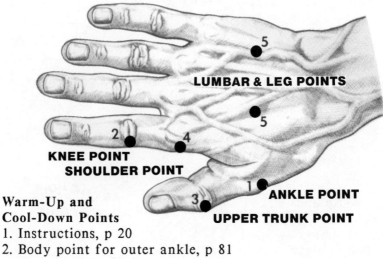

LUMBAR & LEG POINTS

KNEE POINT
SHOULDER POINT

ANKLE POINT

UPPER TRUNK POINT

Warm-Up and
Cool-Down Points
1. Instructions, p 20
2. Body point for outer ankle, p 81

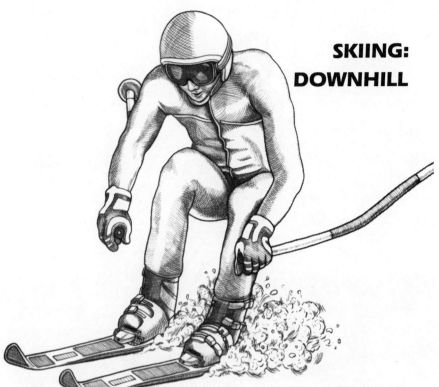

SKIING: DOWNHILL

SKI

PARTICIPANTS	19,490,000	AREAS INJURED		ANKLE	9.7%
INJURIES	125,000	KNEE	26.0%	SHOULDER	7.6%
SPRAINS/STRAINS	45.1%	FINGER	15.8%	U. TRUNK	6.2%

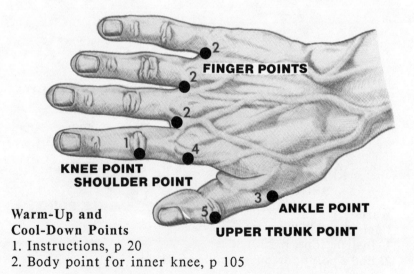

FINGER POINTS

KNEE POINT
SHOULDER POINT

ANKLE POINT

UPPER TRUNK POINT

Warm-Up and
Cool-Down Points
1. Instructions, p 20
2. Body point for inner knee, p 105

SOCCER

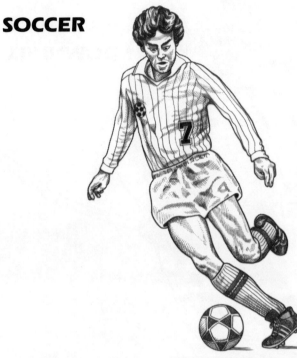

PARTICIPANTS	8,031,000	AREAS INJURED		FINGER	10.4%
INJURIES	342,000	ANKLE	18.1%	FOOT	9.4%
SPRAINS/STRAINS	37.7%	KNEE	13.0%	WRIST	7.1%

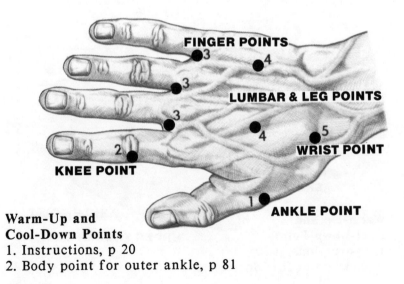

FINGER POINTS
3
4
3
LUMBAR & LEG POINTS
3
4
5
2
WRIST POINT
KNEE POINT
1
ANKLE POINT

**Warm-Up and
Cool-Down Points**
1. Instructions, p 20
2. Body point for outer ankle, p 81

38

SWIMMING

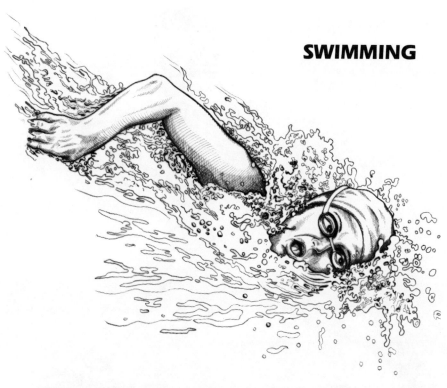

PARTICIPANTS 102,286,000	AREAS INJURED		EAR	9.0%
INJURIES 82,605	TOE	15.3%	FACE	8.8%
SPRAINS/STRAINS 7.3%	HEAD	13.3%	FOOT	5.5%

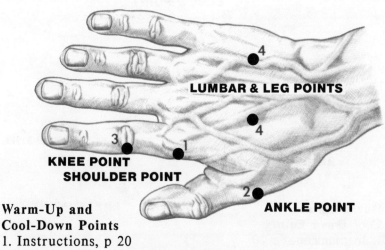

LUMBAR & LEG POINTS

KNEE POINT
SHOULDER POINT

ANKLE POINT

Warm-Up and
Cool-Down Points
1. Instructions, p 20
2. Body point for shoulder, p 129

TENNIS

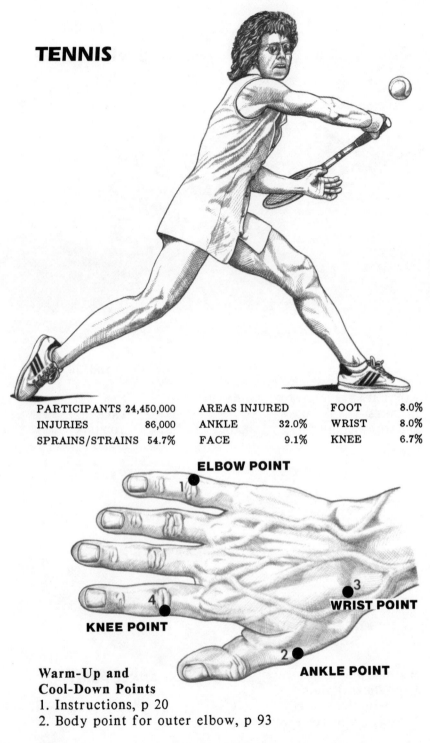

PARTICIPANTS	24,450,000	AREAS INJURED		FOOT	8.0%
INJURIES	86,000	ANKLE	32.0%	WRIST	8.0%
SPRAINS/STRAINS	54.7%	FACE	9.1%	KNEE	6.7%

ELBOW POINT

WRIST POINT

KNEE POINT

ANKLE POINT

**Warm-Up and
Cool-Down Points**
1. Instructions, p 20
2. Body point for outer elbow, p 93

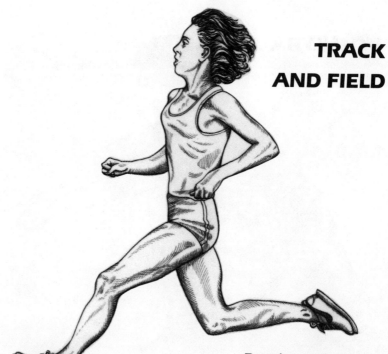

TRACK
AND FIELD

Running and Jogging
PARTICIPANTS 34,274000

PARTICIPANTS	929,725	AREAS INJURED		KNEE	12.8%
INJURIES	196,000	ANKLE	32.2%	L. TRUNK	5.5%
SPRAINS/STRAINS	53.1%	FOOT	14.6%	L. LEG	4.8%

National Federation Handbook 83-84

LUMBAR & LEG POINTS

3

3

2

4

1

KNEE POINT
SHOULDER POINT

ANKLE POINT

Warm-Up and
Cool-Down Points
1. Instructions, p 20
2. Body point for outer ankle, p 81

41

VOLLEYBALL

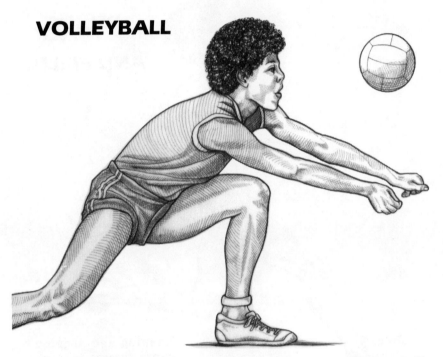

		AREAS INJURED		KNEE	7.9%
PARTICIPANTS	18,365,000				
INJURIES	233,000	FINGER	27.1%	WRIST	7.6%
SPRAINS/STRAINS	51.8%	ANKLE	26.0%	FOOT	6.4%

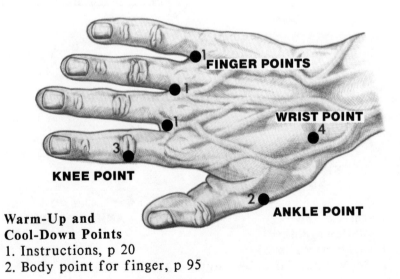

FINGER POINTS

WRIST POINT

KNEE POINT

ANKLE POINT

Warm-Up and Cool-Down Points
1. Instructions, p 20
2. Body point for finger, p 95

WATERSKIING

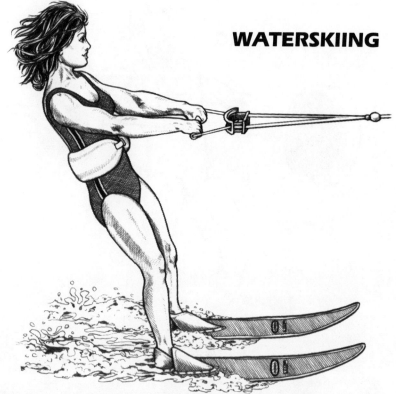

PARTICIPANTS	18,032,000	AREAS INJURED		FACE	8.9%
INJURIES	76,000	HEAD	10.3%	KNEE	8.1%
SPRAINS/STRAINS	24.6%	U. TRUNK	10.1%	FOOT	7.5%

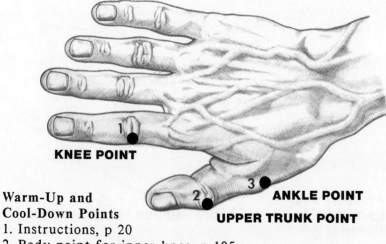

KNEE POINT

ANKLE POINT

UPPER TRUNK POINT

Warm-Up and
Cool-Down Points
1. Instructions, p 20
2. Body point for inner knee, p 105

WEIGHTLIFTING

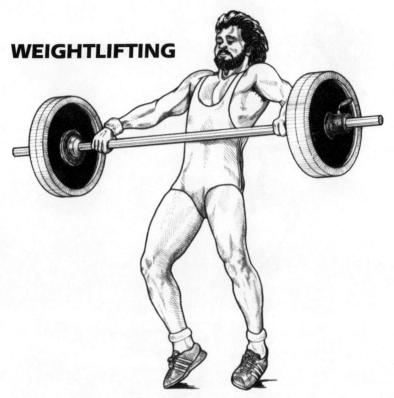

PARTICIPANTS	unknown	AREAS INJURED		TOE	10.7%
INJURIES	126,000	L. TRUNK	14.4%	U. TRUNK	10.5%
SPRAINS/STRAINS	32.5%	FINGER	13.1%	SHOULDER	7.4%

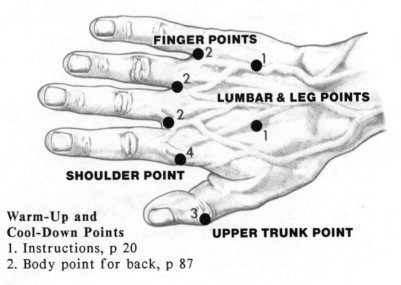

FINGER POINTS

LUMBAR & LEG POINTS

SHOULDER POINT

UPPER TRUNK POINT

Warm-Up and
Cool-Down Points
1. Instructions, p 20
2. Body point for back, p 87

44

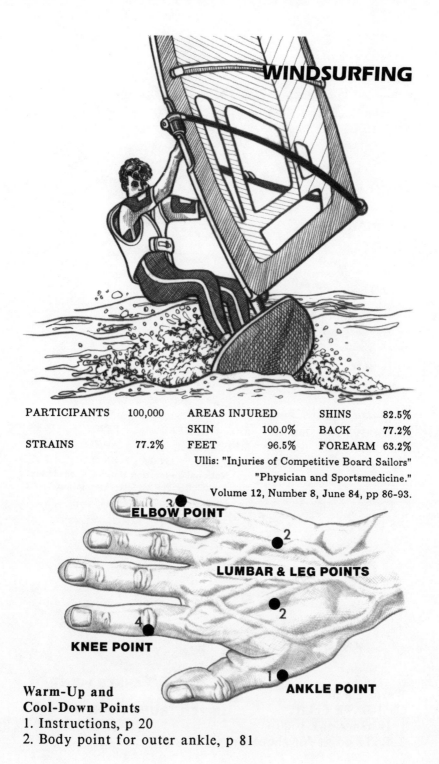

WINDSURFING

PARTICIPANTS	100,000	AREAS INJURED		SHINS	82.5%
		SKIN	100.0%	BACK	77.2%
STRAINS	77.2%	FEET	96.5%	FOREARM	63.2%

Ullis: "Injuries of Competitive Board Sailors"
"Physician and Sportsmedicine."
Volume 12, Number 8, June 84, pp 86-93.

ELBOW POINT 3

2

LUMBAR & LEG POINTS

2

KNEE POINT 4

1 **ANKLE POINT**

Warm-Up and Cool-Down Points
1. Instructions, p 20
2. Body point for outer ankle, p 81

WRESTLING

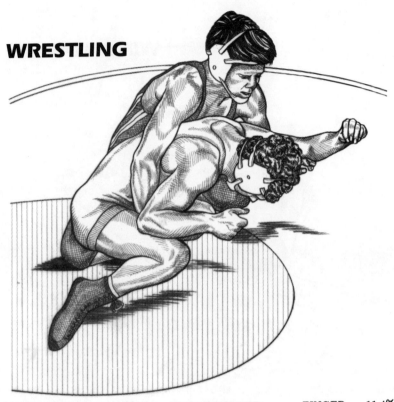

PARTICIPANTS	262,744	AREAS INJURED		FINGER	11.4%
INJURIES	193,000	SHOULDER	12.8%	ANKLE	7.5%
SPRAINS/STRAINS	39.7%	U. TRUNK	11.9%	KNEE	7.1%

National Federation Handbook 83-84 and
National Collegiate Athletic Association 82-83

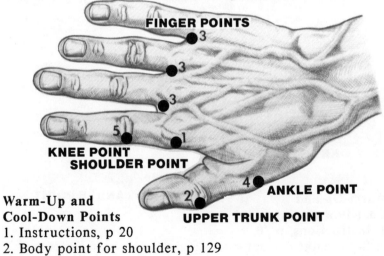

FINGER POINTS

KNEE POINT
SHOULDER POINT

ANKLE POINT

UPPER TRUNK POINT

**Warm-Up and
Cool-Down Points**
1. Instructions, p 20
2. Body point for shoulder, p 129

46

OVER-ALL COOL-DOWN

Wrist Acupressure

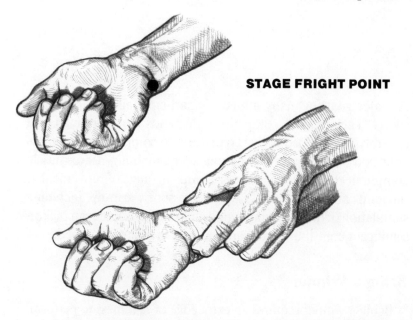

STAGE FRIGHT POINT

Ear Acupressure

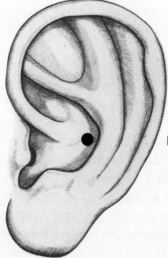

MUSCLE RELAXING POINT

Cool-Down instructions, p 20

Acupressure
Pre-Competition

A major goal for many athletes is participating in competitive sports. The stress of competition demands a well-trained and superbly conditioned body. To perform to competition standards your body needs good circulation, adequate brain-nerve-muscle communication, strong muscles, complete range of movement at the joints and stable joints. An acupressure warm-up, including stimulation of the pre-competition acupressure points, can make a significant contribution towards success in athletic competition.

Being a Winner

Being a winner requires an extra edge or readiness to perform. Stimulation of pre-competition acupressure points can make a significant contribution towards your success by promoting the properly balanced mental and psychological attitudes so frequently reported by winners. In major competitions, the physical capabilities of athletes are likely to be very close, and the true challenge is the mental-psychological one.

Acupressure can produce naturally the proper mental stimulation or relaxation to balance your body. Pre-competition stress is detrimental only in extremes. If the stress level is too low, performance will be uninspired and lacking enthusiasm. Being too anxious, however, creates distress that drains energy and hampers performance. Proper balance produces performance that is both energetic and relaxed. This is peak performance. Stimulating the pre-competition points can turn an *off* day to an *on* day in less than a minute. No other treatment requires less time. Acupressure is the quickest, most effective way to ready yourself for performance.

48

Using the Pre-Competition Points

To fully prepare for a competitive event, use the over-all warm-up points (p 21), the day before competition. Even better, use them on a regular basis, but they are a must the day prior to a big event.

On the day of competition, use the pre-competition points five minutes before you expect to perform to heighten your body's awareness and readiness to respond. Because you want stimulation before competitive situations, use a pinching or jabbing technique on pre-competition points, rather than steady pressure. Simply pinch or jab repeatedly 10 times. For the *Go-Power Point* (p 51), jab firmly, repeatedly and quickly. Relax your breathing. Do not synchronize it with the quick presses. Do visualize yourself beginning, enjoying and winning the event.

Do not repeat stimulation of the pre-competition points until at least 10 minutes have passed or you may find the prolonged stimulation; has a relaxing, sedating effect. The pre-competition points have their greatest effect in short duration events, where quick bursts of energy are required. Because the *Go-Power Point* is in the ear, it can be stimulated periodically during many longer events. Runners, for instance, can easily stimulate this ear acupressure point as they speed along.

Because every athlete is different, you may prefer relaxation rather than stimulation prior to competition. This may be especially true in longer events where endurance is a major factor. If this is the case, refer to the cool-down points (p 47) and use them as part of your pre-competition routine.

The effects of the pre-competition and cool-down points enhance rather than cancel each other. Relaxation and alertness can be very compatible.

Feel free to experiment with any of the points and find what is best for you. However, generally speaking, most athletes will find that using their personal acupressure warm-up, followed by regular stretching or warm-up exercises and topped-off by use of the pre-competition acupressure points, helps them achieve maximum performance in any athletic contest.

> **PRE-COMPETITION
> ACUPRESSURE TECHNIQUE:**
> 1. 10 quick hard pinches or jabs on pre-competition points.
>   - Do both left and right sides, as appropriate.
>   - Breath Deeply.
>   - Visualize the body beginning, enjoying and winning the contest.
> 2. Expect to feel:
>   - Good hurt at the pre-competition points.
>   - More energy and readiness to perform.

PRE-COMPETITION

Body Acupressure

FIGHTING SPIRIT POINT

PRE-COMPETITION

Foot Acupressure

COMPETITIVE EDGE POINT

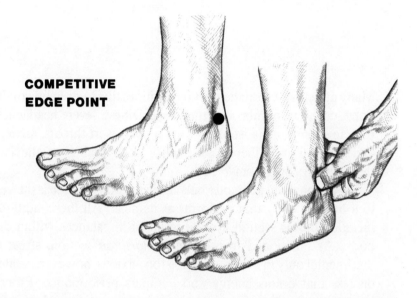

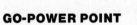

Ear Acupressure

GO-POWER POINT

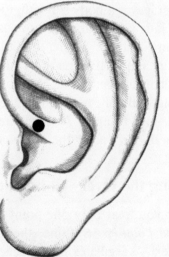

Acupressure
Body
Balancing

Many athletes perform below their abilities due to stressful conditions such as insomnia, appetite loss, dizziness, severe headaches, muscle spasms, exhaustion, common colds, sort throats, anxiety and indigestion. Is there a safe, quick, easy method to alleviate these types of symptoms? Yes!

Ear acupressure promotes balance in the body, which is the key to a healthy body that performs at its peak. All the conditions included in this section are the result of imbalances within the body. As mentioned in the *Pre-Competition* section, stress is detrimental only in extremes. Being too anxious, however, creates distress that drains energy and hampers performance. Proper balance produces performance that is both energetic and relaxed: peak performance.

Likewise, sleep must be balanced to be most effective. Too much leaves a body sluggish; too little leaves the body unrested and fatigued, weakened and susceptible to stress. Appetite also requires balance. Eating too little can be very detrimental to the energy and motivation of an athlete. An over-active appetite can result in unwanted weight that hampers agility, flexibility and strength. By alleviating negative symptoms the body is brought back into balance. Acupressure has been found to do this by naturally producing the proper stimulation or relaxation.

Using the Over-All Balancing Point

If you treat only one point to improve your health, use the *Brain Point* (p 56). Since the brain — specifically the cerebral cortex — regulates all aspects of your body, the *Brain Point* becomes the single most effective over-all treatment point for physical health, emotional balance and mental alertness. It can enhance the results of any other points or acupressure treatment methods.

Regaining Control of Substance Abuse

If you are feeling adverse effects from chemical substances such as alcohol, marijuana, tobacco, cocaine, tranquillizers or anti-depressants, the acupressure points shown under *Substance Abuse Control* (pp 64 to 65) may help reduce the unpleasant symptoms and speed you on your way to better control and more normal functioning.

In substance abuse the respiratory and nervous system seem to be most affected. Thus, the *Lung Point* and *Neurogate Point* are important in the treatment for each substance. Use the additional points for added effectiveness. Acupressure can be effective if used frequently and especially when you feel the urge to take the substance. The points recommended seem to stimulate the body's own natural substances — endorphin, serotonin, cortisone, etc. — so the addictive drug is desired less or not at all.

To make your acupressure treatments more effective:
1. Drink 1 cup of warm water per hour and continue to do so until the urge to take the substance is gone. Drink a cup of water each time before smoking tobacco or marijuana.
2. Eat cooked vegetables, meat and especially romaine lettuce, banana, tofu and wheat germ.
3. Progressively increase aerobic-type exercises, such as brisk walking, rebounding, swimming or biking.

If you feel dependent on or addicted to a substance, it usually takes the following days of abstinence to break the attachment:
Tobacco: 3 days
Alcohol: 5 days
Tranquilizers, Antidepressants, Marijuana or Cocaine: 7 to 14 days

If you are not able to go without the substance for these periods of time or you experience very uncomfortable withdrawal symptoms, please consult a certified acupuncturist. No other treatment has shown itself to be so effective, pleasant, safe and quick.

Treating for Balance

For most conditions, use ear acupressure as soon as you are aware of the symptoms. Simply follow the directions given. Repeat as often as needed or as desired.

For chronic conditions, extended stimulation of the ear acupressure point may be more effective than the usual 1 minute application. As much as 5 to 10 minutes per treatment is not excessive. In fact, it seems impossible to over-do ear acupressure. If you prolong the treatment, you can expect increased relaxation and reduced symptoms, discomfort and pain. For these extended treatments, deep, synchronized breathing is very important. Visualize the symptoms leaving your body as you apply pressure and exhale, and health being restored as you relax pressure and inhale.

Chronic conditions, such as migraine headaches, prolonged indigestion, depression or menstrual problems, may take months of repeated treatments to significantly improve. Though acupressure can quickly reduce pain and swelling, it make take a while to correct the body chemistry and rebuild the health of an over-stressed and weak body. It usually takes years for an unhealthy condition to develop, so give your body some time to repair itself.

Many health care professionals have found acupressure effective for the conditions mentioned in this book. If several days to a week of repeated treatment does not improve the condition, you may wish to seek medical advice. Be sure to follow the suggestions for maintaining health (p 12) to speed your healing.

Acupressure does not supercede good medical service, but in emergency situations it can be used immediately while waiting for medical help. Also it can safely be used in conjunction with other treatments.

BODY BALANCING
ACUPRESSURE TECHNIQUE:
1. Apply firm pressure on right ear point for 1 minute: 5 seconds on - 5 seconds off.
   - Maintain skin contact.
   - Exhale while pressing ear point.
   - Visualize enhanced body balance health.
2. Expect to feel:
   - Hot stinging sensation at the ear point during pressure.
   - Greater body balance and health.
3. Apply pressure to left ear for added effectiveness.

NOTE: Three of the ear points (*Subcortex:* p 58, *Ovary:* p 60 and *Excitation:* p 60) are inside the lower ear fold (the anti-tragus area). The *Throat Point*, p 65, is inside the forward ear fold (the tragus area). Apply a squeezing pressure with thumb and finger to these four points. They are noted by a circle around the point and an asterisk (*) by the name.

OVER-ALL BALANCE

Try this! The brain point is the over-all point to maximize health and performance. Use it alone or along with any of the other points. Use it as often as you wish.

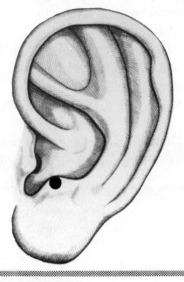

BRAIN POINT

APPETITE BALANCE

Try this for: Loss of appetite, compulsive eating, under- and over-weight conditions.

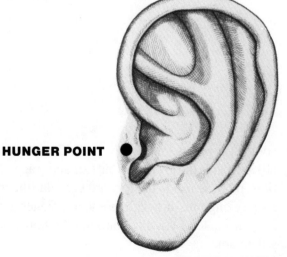

HUNGER POINT

BODY BALANCE instructions, p 55

DIGESTION BALANCE

Try this for: Alleviating indigestion, nausea, belching or heart burn.

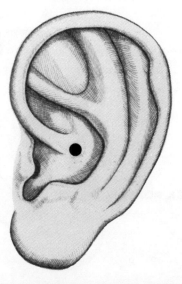

STOMACH POINT

ELIMINATION BALANCE

Try this for: Relief of constipation or diarrhea.

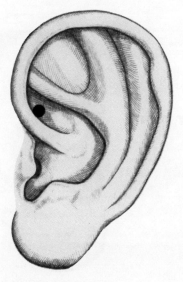

LARGE INTESTINE POINT

FAINTING CONTROL

Try this for: Fainting, insomnia and neurotic symptoms.

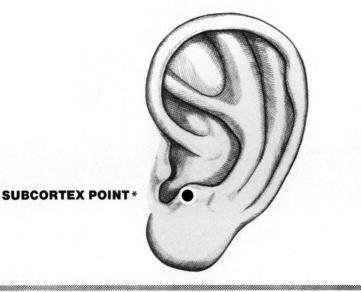

SUBCORTEX POINT *

FRACTURE HEALING

Try this: To speed the healing of bone fractures and for dizziness and kidney injury.

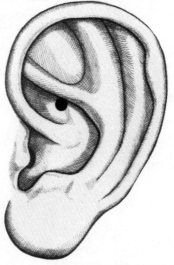

KIDNEY POINT

58

BODY BALANCE instructions, p 55

HEADACHE RELIEF

Try this for: Alleviating headaches and symptoms of concusion.

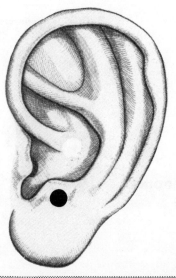

HEADACHE POINT

INFLAMMATION CONTROL

Try this for: All inflammatory conditions, as well as irritated and swollen joints, muscles and tendons. This point can also be used for allergies, common cold, fever and shortness of breath.

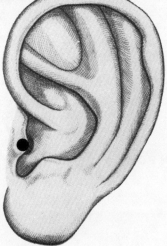

ADRENAL POINT

59

MENSTRUAL BALANCE

Try this for: Alleviating painful, irregular menstruation.

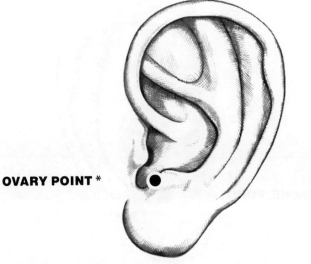

OVARY POINT *

MOOD ELEVATION

Try this for: Alleviating depression, apathy, emotional withdrawal and excessive sleeping.

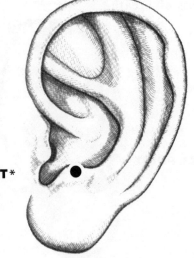

EXCITATION POINT*

BODY BALANCE instructions, p 55

MOTION BALANCE

Try this for: Alleviating jet lag, car and sea sickness.

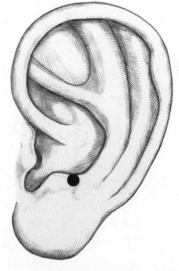

OCCIPUT POINT

MUSCLE BALANCE

Try this for: Relaxation (muscle relaxing point) and weakness (spleen point).

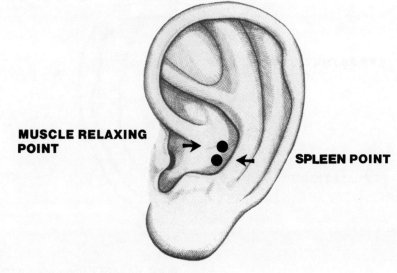

MUSCLE RELAXING POINT

SPLEEN POINT

61

PAIN CONTROL

Try this for: Reducing any body pain and anxiety.

NEUROGATE POINT

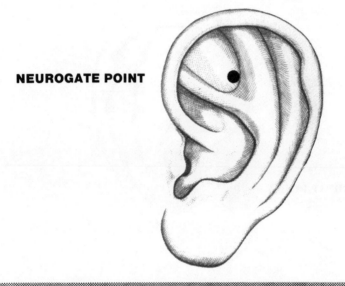

PERSPIRATION BALANCE

Try this for: Regulating excessive or slight perspiration.

SYMPATHETIC POINT

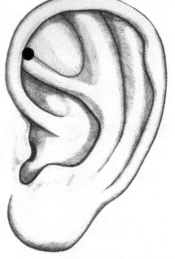

BODY BALANCE instructions, p 55

SCIATIC RELIEF

Try this for: Relieving sciatica.

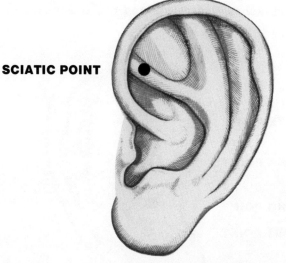

SCIATIC POINT

SHOCK RELIEF

Try this: To reduce the symptoms of shock: faintness, skin pale, cold and clammy, pulse rapid and weak, breath shallow. Requires immediate care by a physician.

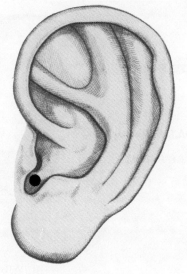

STEROID POINT

SUBSTANCE ABUSE CONTROL

Try this for all Substance Abuse Control: To reduce withdrawal symtoms such as abdominal cramps, shakes, diarrhea, irritability, fatigue, bone aches, wheezing, rhinitis, headaches, depression and eye tearing.

Alcohol

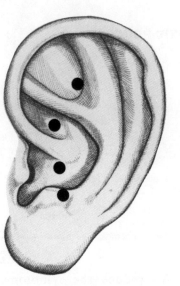

NEUROGATE POINT

DRUNK POINT

LUNG POINT
OCCIPUT POINT

Tobacco,
Marijuana and
Cocaine

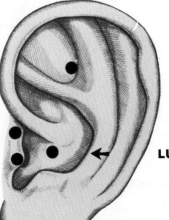

NEUROGATE POINT

THROAT POINT
ADRENAL POINT

LUNG POINT

BODY BALANCE instructions, p 55

64

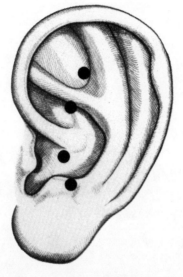

NEUROGATE POINT

KIDNEY POINT

LUNG POINT

OCCIPUT POINT

THROAT HEALTH

Try this for: Alleviating sore throat, laryngitis, hoarseness and tonsilitis.

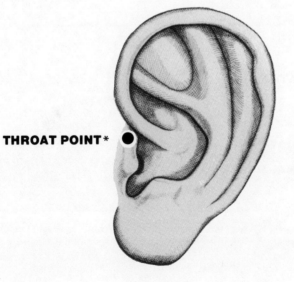

THROAT POINT *

2

ACUPRESSURE FOR SPRAINS AND STRAINS

Athletic
Injuries

The human body is a miraculous piece of engineering. The proper functioning of bone and muscle allows athletes to achieve peak performance in sports and competition. But even a body that performs well must still cope with a great deal of physical stress. Some of the over 200 bones in the body experience thousands of pounds of pressure per square inch while performing the simple action of walking. The stress of training can cause certain bones in the athlete's body to build and strengthen. However, no matter how well-developed the skeleton is, it takes muscles to move those bones.

More than 600 muscles contribute to an athlete performing well. It has been estimated that an athlete's muscles probably do the equivalent of loading 50,000 pounds onto a 4-foot-high shelf during a good workout or sports competition. If all the work the muscles do could be co-ordinated in one direction at one time, any athlete could lift the weight of a semi-truck.

In sports, the flexibility and strength of muscles are as important as strong joints. Muscles are responsible for moving every part of the body. The brain has voluntary control over more than 425 muscles. When the body performs properly, the brain sends messages via the nerves telling the muscles how hard and when to contract and to relax. However, when a muscle is injured, messages of pain and discomfort are sent to the brain and interfere with performance. Then the body must repair itself before it can function efficiently. Millions of athletes receive muscle injuries. In fact, the U.S. government estimates there are about 15 million muscle injuries a year.

In addition to well-developed bones and muscles, several other factors effect optimum athletic health and performance. These include good circulation and respiration, stable joint structure, muscles that are flexible as well as strong, and efficient nerve communication between the brain and the muscles. These body parts and systems are all closely interrelated and failure of any single part of the body greatly hampers ability to train and compete.

Each year over 10 million athletes are injured seriously enough to require medical attention. The major injuries include sprains, strains, bruises, scrapes, cuts and bone fractures. Of all these injuries, by far the most common are sprains and strains. In football, for example, over one-third of all injuries are sprains and strains; in basketball, over half are of these two types.

Since sprains and strains are the most common types of injury, any athlete serious about training and competing, benefits from understanding these injuries. Such knowledge enables an athlete to cope with these problems correctly, recover in the minimum amount of time and, hopefully, prevent them from recurring. Before learning how to treat sprains and strains, look briefly at what happens in the body when these injuries occur.

Spraining a Ligament

What is a sprain? A sprain occurs when a ligament is stretched beyond its capacity and is torn. Ligaments are found at the joints. All ligaments contribute to the body's stability and potential for balanced movement by holding the bones together securely at the joints.

What happens when ligaments are injured? Some or all of the many fibers of the ligament tear and nerve endings are injured. A message is immediately sent to the brain relaying sharp pain at the joint. Next, blood and tissue fluids containing protein flow into the damaged area, causing the ligament and the joint area to swell. Then blood clots create a weak ligament scar composed of protein fibers. These new fibers grow, connecting the torn tissue (much as new bone tissue heals a fracture). It takes time for the fibers to connect and the damaged nerves to regenerate and gain strength. Finally, the scar may become as strong as the original tissue and the ligament is renewed.

Ligament sprains are categorized as mild, moderate or severe. Most sprains are mild to moderate tears of the ligament. These are the ones you can successfully treat. The healing process for mild to moderate sprains usually takes from 2 to 4 weeks, depending on how many ligament fibers were torn.

Severe sprains take the longest to heal because they may rip all the fibers of the ligament and leave the injured part totally unable to move. In this case surgery may be suggested. Thus, for severe sprains consultation with a physician is advisable.

Since the joints and ligaments in an athlete's body must withstand tremendous amounts of constant stress and pressure, it is not surprising that many are injured. The most commonly injured joints, for all sports, are finger and ankle.

Straining a Muscle

What is a strain? A strain occurs when a muscle or a tendon is stretched or stressed beyond its capacity and is torn or pulled.

The degree of possible injury to a muscle increases as the amount of stress increases. A muscle strain often occurs in response to quick changes of the tension within the muscle. Sudden bursts of speed as in charging the net in tennis, running for a touchdown in football, sprinting in track or over-exerting in aerobics are events that can cause muscle strain.

Muscles are made of hundreds of fibers about the thickness of a human hair. Strains occur anywhere within the muscle: either in the fleshy body part or at its junction with the tendon (which connects the muscle to bone).

When a muscle tears, blood and tissue fluids accumulate in the area of the injury and may cause swelling of the muscle and discoloration of the skin. The muscle becomes stiff and the joint loses its full range-of-motion. Then a process of healing similar to that for ligament sprains occurs, with new tissue forming a scar connecting torn muscle fibers.

As with ligament sprains, muscle strains are divided into 3 categories: mild, moderate and severe — depending basically on how many of the muscle fibers are torn. With a severe muscle tear you probably would not be able to contract the muscle at all. You would not be able to move the injured body part. Severe strains may at times require surgery to help speed the healing process, so the guidance of a physician is strongly advised.

Most muscle strains, however, are mild to moderate tears and may be successfully treated with acupressure. The healing time for muscle strains can be less than that needed for ligament sprains because muscles have better circulation than ligaments. Therefore, they have a greater supply of blood protein to form scar tissue over the torn fibers. Healing takes from several days to many weeks, depending on the number of torn fibers. For mild strains use of the muscle is possible without pain after a few days. For moderate strains healing may take longer with pain and weakness persisting for 2 to 4 weeks, or longer.

Straining a Tendon

The approximately 1,000 tendons of the body are also subject to strains. Tendons attach muscles to bones and are made of strong, rope-like fibers that do not contract. A tendon can be strained in the same way a muscle is strained, that is by a sudden, sharp movement during tension.

More frequently, however, tendon strains or tendinitis are an inflammatory condition resulting from chronic overuse and aggravated by three factors. First, tendons are more exposed than muscles in the sense that they come into contact with bones, ligaments and other tendons. This contact can result in friction that leads to irritation and microtearing. As inflammation progresses, swelling tissues constrict blood flow, limit movement and cause pain.

Second, when muscles are exercised strenuously over an extended period of time, they tend to maintain a degree of contraction even at rest. The tendons are then under constant tension. This in turn leads to microtrauma and inflammation. Third, frequent repetition of a body movement with insufficient rest can cause tendon strain from overuse. A subsequent period of inactivity can allow the formation of adhesions, microscars within the tendon tissue. The body should be reintroduced to athletic stress gently. Flexibility, range of movement and strength need to be built to your previous levels gradually, or tendons can be re-injured.

When a tendon has been injured the body heals the torn fibers with scar tissue much as it heals ligament sprains and muscle strains. However, healing tendon strains may require extended periods of rest to avoid further irritation. Non-stressful activity during healing is important to maintain circulation and flexibility in the area, but movement must be gradual and should not continue when acute or excessive pain is present. Sudden or stressful movements can re-tear previously injured fibers. Healing may take from 2 to 4 weeks, or longer.

Healing Your Injuries

If you are injured, the responsibility for determining what to do is yours, unless you are unconscious. You must decide whether to seek medical assistance and what form that help will take. There are now many licensed medical practitioners available for consultation, including medical doctors, acupuncturists, chiropractors and physical therapists who specialize in the treatment of athletic injuries.

The common goal of all qualified individuals treating athletic injuries is to assess the extent of your injury, to provide immediate care, to reduce pain, swelling and inflammation, and to promote the best and fastest healing possible. Although different techniques and treatments may be used, all medical practitioners emphasize the importance of proper care of the injury until the ligament, muscle or tendon tears have completely healed.

To assure yourself of good treatment for your injuries, rapid return of strength, flexibility and range-of-movement, it is essential to play an active, informed role in your healing process. Make yourself aware of all the treatment possibilities, seek sound medical advice when necessary and choose the methods of healing most appropriate for you.

Acupressure Treatment

Whether or not you choose to see a licensed medical practitioner, you should immediately begin treatment of a sprain or strain. If your injury produces significant swelling within the first few hours, it is wise to seek professional advice. If you have constant pain from your injury, it is wise to seek professional advice. When in doubt, seek professional advice.

Immediate Care

Using RICE

The commonly accepted first aid treatment is Rest, Ice, Compression and Elevation. The word *RICE* is a convenient way to remember these treatment steps. The purpose of using *RICE* is to reduce pain, prevent further swelling and bleeding, and stop damage of ligament, muscle and/or tendon fibers.

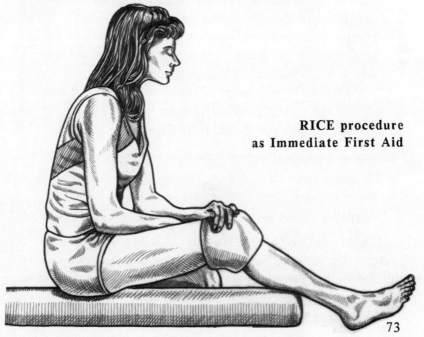

RICE procedure
as Immediate First Aid

Rest: Stop using the part of your body that is injured, it needs rest to heal properly. Restrict movement during the first 24 to 48 hours. Further activity or exercise could cause pain and additional tearing of ligament, muscle or tendon fibers.

Ice: Apply ice to the injured area. Use an ice bag or cloth to contain the ice. Place a towel over the injured area; do not apply ice directly to the skin as it can cause damage and pain. Leave ice on an injury for a maximum of 15 minutes at a time. This procedure may be repeated as needed, but not more frequently than every 2 to 3 hours, for 2 to 3 days. *Avoid using ice too long or too frequently as it may cause frostbite or tissue damage.* Ice causes constriction of the blood vessels and helps to slow down the swelling that often begins the moment an injury occurs. Swelling is caused by accumulation of blood and body fluids in the tissue surrounding torn fibers. These excess fluids can increase recovery time.

Compression: After removing the ice, wrap the injury with an elastic bandage. Do not wrap too tightly because circulation to the injured area may be cut off. Cramping, numbness and increased pain are signs that blood flow has been reduced too much. If you experience any of these symptoms, remove the bandage immediately.

Elevate: Whenever possible during the first 24 hours, elevate the injured area above your heart. This permits gravity to drain excess fluid from the injured area.

If your injury is still painful after 72 hours, it is important to increase circulation. Heat may be recommended and can be applied by hot towels, a hot bath or a heating pad. If pain or swelling increase, discontinue heat until later.

Treating with Hand and Ear Acupressure

An acupressure treatment for injury follows the general guidelines given in the *Acupressure Technique* section (pp 7 to 13). You may treat yourself with acupressure as often as you like. As long as the treatment produces a lessening of pain it is beneficial to continue. You cannot harm your body by using acupressure too long or too frequently. Each time you treat yourself, you may stop when you feel a significant reduction of pain. Injury to any part of your body can produce shock and trauma all through your body. You may enhance the treatment of your injury by combining it with an appropriate *Body Balancing* treatment (pp 53 to 65).

Allow yourself to relax and be as comfortable as possible. If a friend graciously offers to treat you, please accept. It helps you to relax more completely. For some injuries — such as a sprained wrist or finger — help from a friend may be essential.

After beginning your treatment with the *RICE* procedure, continue with the hand acupressure technique. Carefully locate the proper point and follow the directions given.

Visualizing the pain leaving your injury can improve your treatment. Your attitudes and emotions effect your body chemistry. As you change your attitude to one of health and relaxation, your body heals more easily.

The healing process for sprains and strains usually causes injured parts to become swollen and stiff. After 2 to 3 days, gentle movement of the injury aids circulation and eases stiffness; this is especially true during acupressure treatments. While pressure is applied to the hand points, gently move your injured body part.

If you feel the *good hurt* during hand acupressure but still have pain, proceed with ear acupressure. Follow the steps given. If pain persists, proceed to *Continuing Care.* Be patient and relax as you continue your treatment.

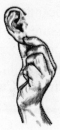

HAND ACUPRESSURE TECHNIQUE:

1. Apply firm pressure on the point for 1 minute: 5 seconds on - 5 seconds off.
   - Apply pressure to hand on side opposite the injury.
   - Maintain skin contact.
   - Visualize pain leaving the injured area while exhaling forcefully.
   - Gently move the injured part if not too painful.
2. Expect to feel:
   - Strong, dull or aching sensation at the pressure point: *good hurt*.
   - Reduction of pain in the injury.
3. If pain is not significantly reduced:
   - Check that pressure on the point was applied correctly and repeat procedure.
   - Repeat procedure to other hand.
   - Proceed to use Ear Acupressure.

EAR ACUPRESSURE TECHNIQUE:

1. Apply firm pressure on point for 1 minute: 5 seconds on - 5 seconds off.
   - Apply pressure to ear on same side as injury.
   - Maintain skin contact.
   - Visualize pain leaving the injured area while exhaling forcefully.
   - Gently move the injured part if not too painful.
2. Expect to feel:
   - Hot stinging sensation at the ear point during pressure.
   - Reduction of pain in the injury.
3. If pain is not significantly reduced:
   - Check that pressure on the point was applied correctly and repeat procedure.
   - Repeat procedure on other ear.
   - Proceed to Continuing Care.

Continuing Care

These body acupressure techniques are slightly different from others because there are no precise acupressure points. If you have injured your right ankle, treatment of the same spot on the uninjured left ankle will benefit the injured ankle. Very simply, this is because your nervous system connects every part of your body — especially the corresponding left/right parts.

Gently explore your injury to find the exact point of most pain. Find the corresponding point on your uninjured side. Follow the directions to apply body acupressure to that point or points. If you have correctly located the corresponding point, you will feel the *good hurt* sensation.

If pain still persists after completing these procedures, you may refer to the ear acupressure steps for *Inflammation Control* (p 59), *Pain Control* (p 62) or any other balancing points that seem appropriate. These *Continuing Care* techniques may be applied daily or as frequently as you wish, until your injury is pain-free even during training or play.

Prevention

These body acupressure points are located at the site of the injury. To avoid pain or aggravation of your injury, do not use these points until your injury is pain-free at rest, which is often 48 to 72 hours after injury. Absence of significant pain is the major indicator that lets you know when your injury is healed sufficiently to sustain stress. This applies whether the source of the stress is treatment directly to the injured area or physical activity.

After any acupressure treatment, pain and discomfort may be relieved and then return temporarily. Pain may even increase for a short time. This is a natural part of the healing process. It indicates that the healing and rebuilding of torn tissue is in process but is not yet complete. This is a stage that may require patience. To treat yourself right, be sure your injury is relatively pain-free at rest for at least 2 days. After that time, you may add these *Prevention* techniques to your *Continuing Care* program.

Using the *Prevention* body acupressure points strengthens areas of recent or chronic injury, and also areas of high risk to injury by your sport. Healing is aided by increased circulation, and by enhanced brain-nerve-muscle communication to the injured area. As part of the *Continuing Care* program, *Prevention* may be used as frequently as you wish. Simply follow the directions.

Once your injury has healed, body acupressure on the appropriate points helps prevent recurrence by strengthening the injured area. Therefore, the *Prevention* acupressure points for a recent, chronic or high-risk injury area are important to include in your acupressure warm-up routine. For added effectiveness, you may use these points on a daily basis. Treat yourself with acupressure as much as you like.

CONTINUING CARE
ACUPRESSURE TECHNIQUE:
1. Locate acupressure points:
   - Gently explore injured area to find the most pain.
   - Find the corresponding area on non-injured side of body.
2. Apply very firm pressure to non-injured side for 1 minute: 5 seconds on - 5 seconds off.
   - Gently more injured area as pressure is applied.
   - Visualize the body part stronger and more flexible as you exhale.
3. Expect to feel:
   - Tenderness or dull ache, good hurt, if correct point has been located.
   - Reduction of pain in the injury.
4. If pain is not significantly reduced:
   - Check location of the point and repeat procedure.
   - Consider treatment by physician/acupuncturist/chiropractor.

PREVENTION ACUPRESSURE TECHNIQUE:

1. Apply firm pressure to left body point for 1 minute: 5 seconds on - 5 seconds off; repeat for right body point.
   - Move opposite part as pressure is applied.
   - Visualize the ligaments, muscles and tendons stronger and more flexible as you exhale.
2. Expect to feel:
   - Good hurt at acupressure point.
   - Greater flexibility, strength and stability in the area.

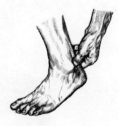

NOTE: The healing times listed for each of the following injuries are estimated according to conventional Western treatments. These times may be greatly reduced by the correct use of acupressure.

ANKLE SPRAIN: outer

ANTERIOR TALOFIBULAR LIGAMENT SPRAIN

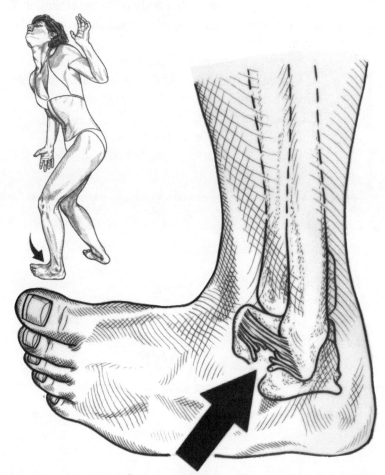

Causes:	Forcefully stepping down on a turned-in foot.
Effects:	Mild or moderate tearing of ligament fibers between lateral ankle bone and foot bone.
Symptoms:	Tenderness, pain, swelling, joint weakness and instability.
Major Sports:	Badminton, Baseball, Basketball, Football, Tennis and Volleyball.
Healing Time:	Mild Sprain: 1 to 2 weeks. Moderate Sprain: about 2 to 4 weeks.

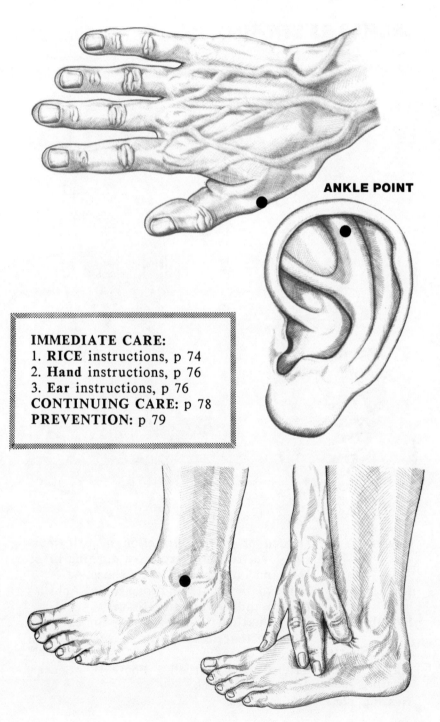

ANKLE POINT

IMMEDIATE CARE:
1. **RICE** instructions, p 74
2. **Hand** instructions, p 76
3. **Ear** instructions, p 76
CONTINUING CARE: p 78
PREVENTION: p 79

ACHILLES STRAIN

ACHILLES TENDINITIS

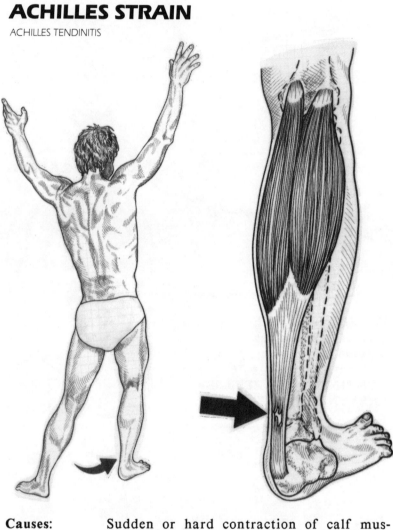

Causes:	Sudden or hard contraction of calf muscles, overtraining, excessive turning-in of foot and improperly fitting shoes.
Effects:	Mild to moderate microtears in Achilles tendon and surrounding tissue.
Symptoms:	Inflammation, swelling and pain early in the day that lessen with movement, then increase later.
Major Sports:	Baseball, Basketball, Football, Soccer, Squash and Track.
Healing Time:	2 to 6 weeks.

82

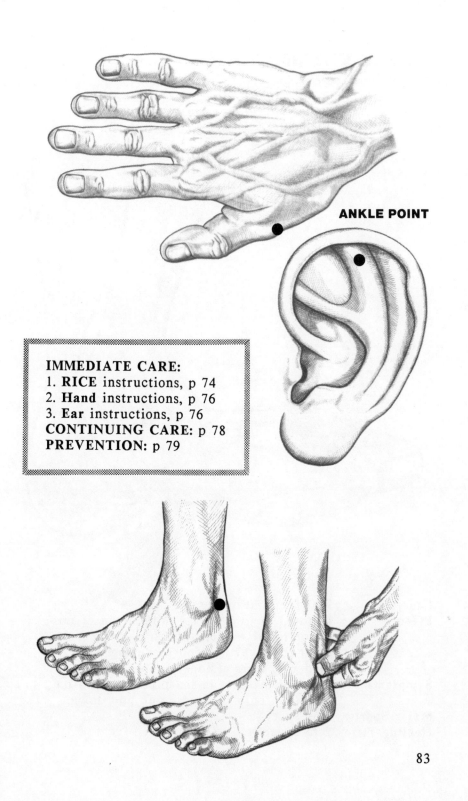

ANKLE POINT

IMMEDIATE CARE:
1. **RICE** instructions, p 74
2. **Hand** instructions, p 76
3. **Ear** instructions, p 76
CONTINUING CARE: p 78
PREVENTION: p 79

ANKLE STRAIN: inner

POSTERIOR TIBIAL TENDINITIS

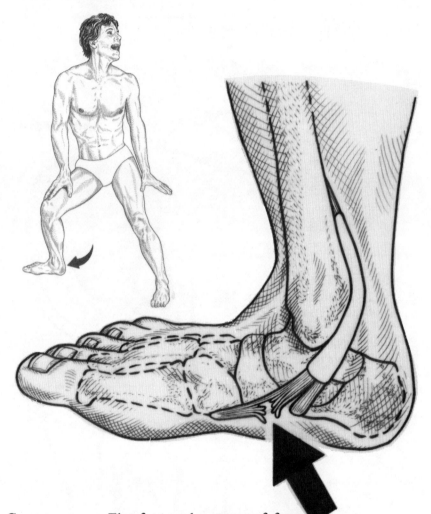

Causes:	Flat feet and overuse of feet.
Effects:	Gradual (4 to 6 weeks) mild strain of posterior tibial tendon (attaches to the navicular bone at midfoot) causing mild to moderate tears of inner foot tendon.
Symptoms:	Gradual increase in sharp pain at midfoot, results in pain if jumping up and down.
Major Sports:	Any sport.
Healing Time:	2 to 3 weeks.

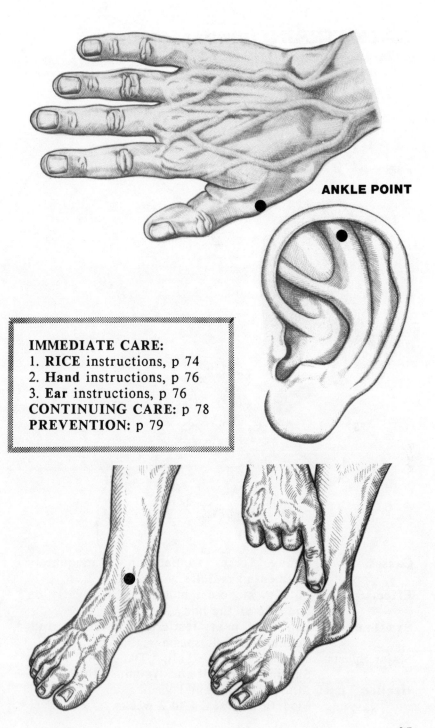

ANKLE POINT

IMMEDIATE CARE:
1. **RICE** instructions, p 74
2. **Hand** instructions, p 76
3. **Ear** instructions, p 76
CONTINUING CARE: p 78
PREVENTION: p 79

BACK STRAIN: lumbar

QUADRATUS LUMBORUM MUSCLE STRAIN

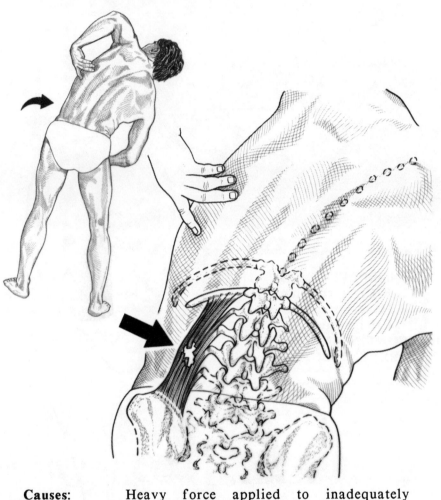

Causes:	Heavy force applied to inadequately warmed-up muscles.
Effects:	Mild to moderate muscle tears, usually on one side of the body.
Symttoms:	Localized pain, tenderness, swelling and, possibly, muscle spasm.
Major Sports:	Baseball, Basketball, Dancing, Figure Skating, Football and Weight-lifting.
Healing Time:	Mild Strain: about 1 week.
	Moderate Strain: 1 to 2 weeks.

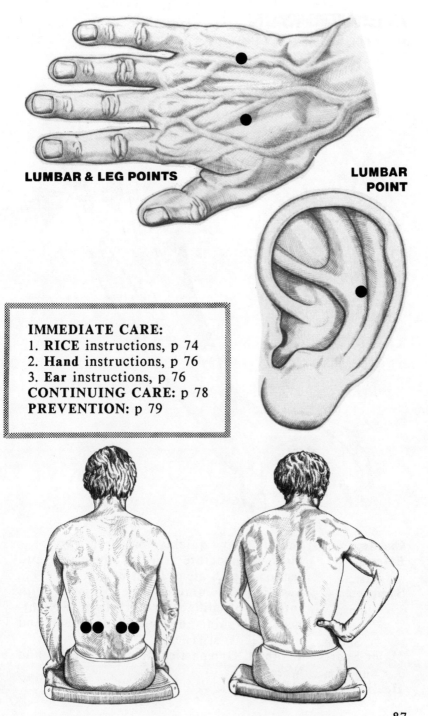

LUMBAR & LEG POINTS

LUMBAR POINT

IMMEDIATE CARE:
1. **RICE** instructions, p 74
2. **Hand** instructions, p 76
3. **Ear** instructions, p 76
CONTINUING CARE: p 78
PREVENTION: p 79

ELBOW SPRAIN

MEDIAL COLLATERAL LIGAMENT SPRAIN

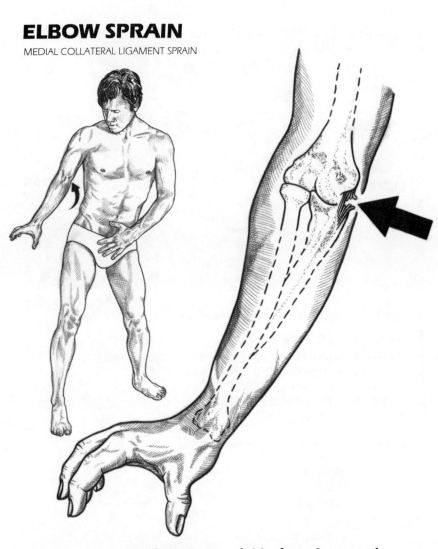

Causes:	Having elbow quickly forced outwards.
Effects:	Mild to moderate tears of ligaments and tendon sheath along front of elbow.
Symptoms:	Swelling 30 minutes after injury, with internal bleeding and a feeling of tightness and pain, and with both inner and outer elbow stiffness.
Major Sports:	Football, Gymnastics, Hockey, Javelin and Wrestling.
Healing Time:	2 to 4 weeks.

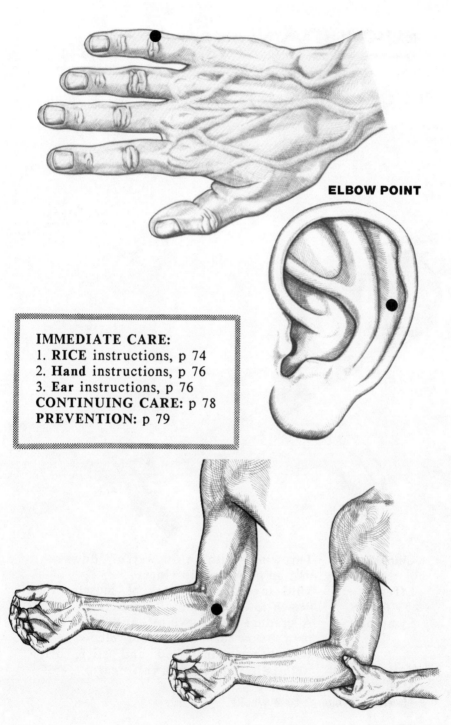

ELBOW POINT

IMMEDIATE CARE:
1. **RICE** instructions, p 74
2. **Hand** instructions, p 76
3. **Ear** instructions, p 76
CONTINUING CARE: p 78
PREVENTION: p 79

89

ELBOW STRAIN: inner

Little League Pitcher's Elbow

INNER FOREARM FLEXOR MUSCLE STRAIN

Causes:	Throwing with a powerful downward motion of wrist and fingers.
Effects:	Mild to moderate tears of muscles that attach to inner knob of elbow.
Symptoms:	A gradual (over several days) build-up of pain below or on knob of elbow. Arm will become inflamed and stiff, often with pain radiating down forearm.
Major Sports:	Baseball.
Healing Time:	2 to 3 weeks.

90

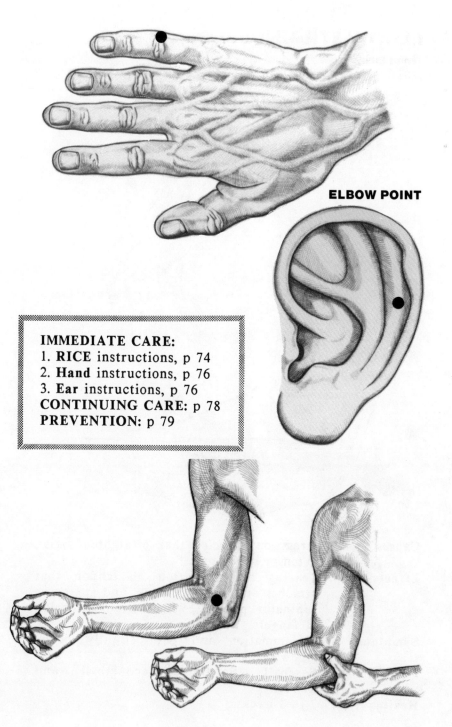

ELBOW POINT

IMMEDIATE CARE:
1. **RICE** instructions, p 74
2. **Hand** instructions, p 76
3. **Ear** instructions, p 76
CONTINUING CARE: p 78
PREVENTION: p 79

ELBOW STRAIN: outer

Tennis Elbow

LATERAL HUMERAL EPICONDYLITIS

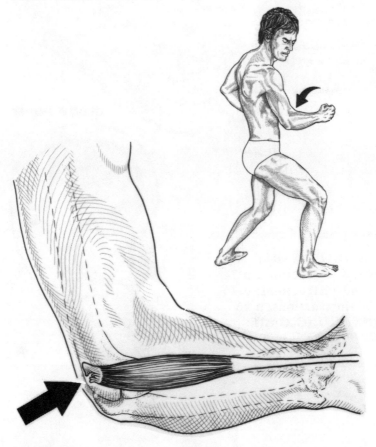

Causes:	Stress on muscles that straighten wrist, extensor supinators.
Effects:	Tearing and irritation of tendon that attaches to outer elbow and extensor supinator muscles, which allow extension of fingers.
Symptoms:	Inflammation and pain slightly below elbow crease.
Major Sports:	Baseball, Bowling, Racquetball and Tennis.
Healing Time:	2 to 3 weeks.

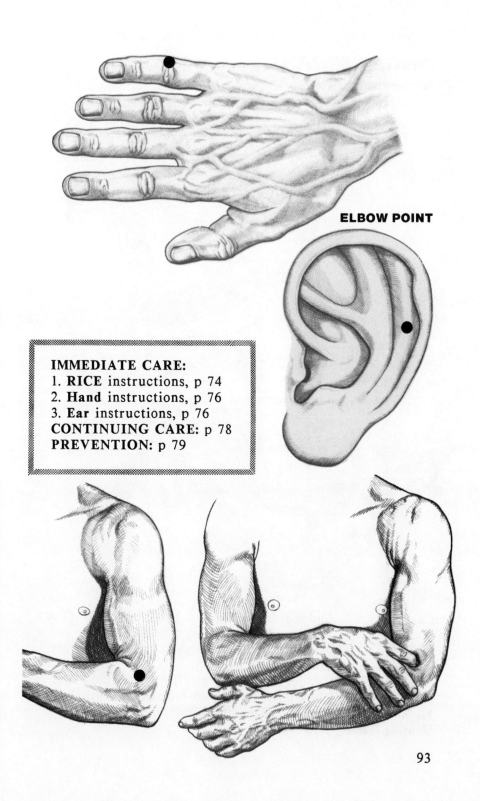

ELBOW POINT

IMMEDIATE CARE:
1. **RICE** instructions, p 74
2. **Hand** instructions, p 76
3. **Ear** instructions, p 76
CONTINUING CARE: p 78
PREVENTION: p 79

FINGER SPRAIN

Jammed Finger

PROXIMAL INTERPHALANGEAL JOINT
COLLATERAL LIGAMENT SPRAIN

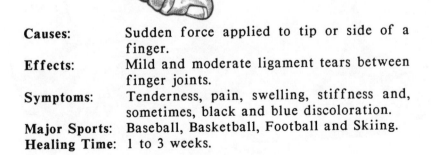

Causes:	Sudden force applied to tip or side of a finger.
Effects:	Mild and moderate ligament tears between finger joints.
Symptoms:	Tenderness, pain, swelling, stiffness and, sometimes, black and blue discoloration.
Major Sports:	Baseball, Basketball, Football and Skiing.
Healing Time:	1 to 3 weeks.

94

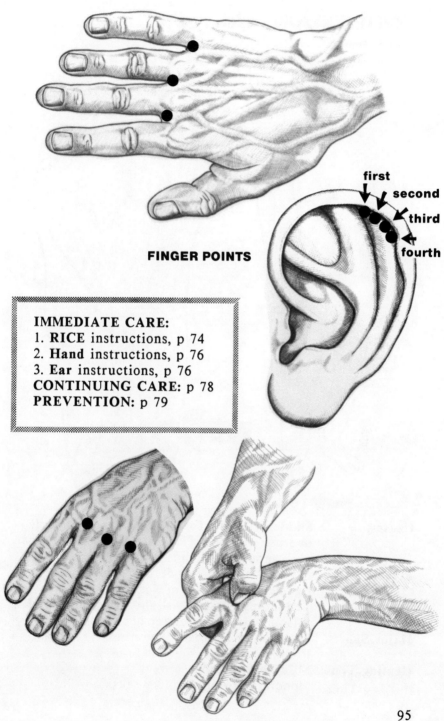

FINGER POINTS

first
second
third
fourth

IMMEDIATE CARE:
1. **RICE** instructions, p 74
2. **Hand** instructions, p 76
3. **Ear** instructions, p 76
CONTINUING CARE: p 78
PREVENTION: p 79

95

FOOT SPRAIN: arch

PLANTAR FASCITIS

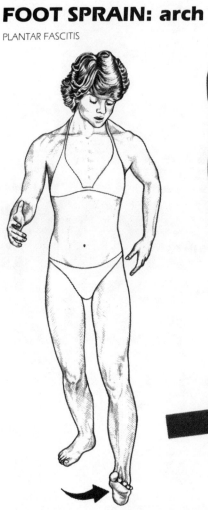
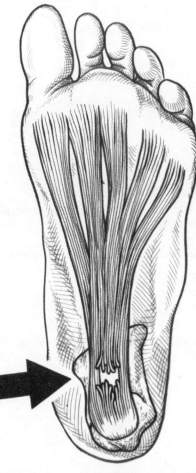

Causes:	Sudden hard force on heel, chronic overuse of foot, flat feet, shoes with no arch support and shoes with stiff soles.
Effects:	Partial mild to moderate tears in arch ligament on bottom of foot.
Symptoms:	Tenderness, pain, slight swelling and inflammation just under heel bone.
Major Sports:	Basketball, Football, Running, Track and Field.
Healing Time:	Mild Sprain: about 1 week. Moderate Sprain: 2 to 3 weeks.

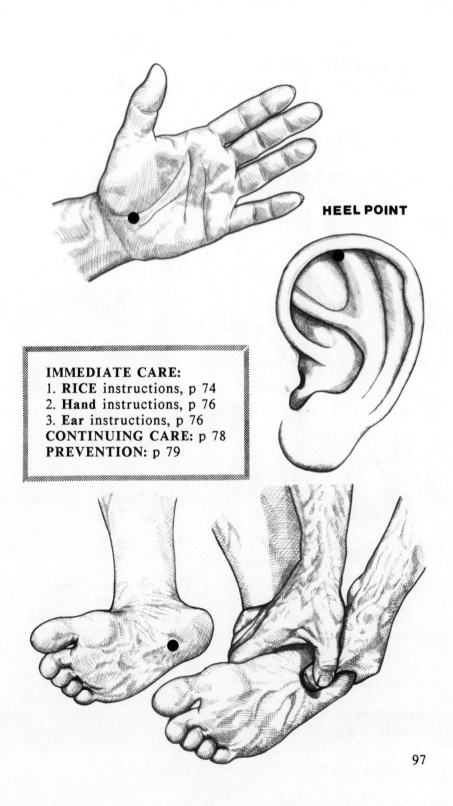

HEEL POINT

IMMEDIATE CARE:
1. **RICE** instructions, p 74
2. **Hand** instructions, p 76
3. **Ear** instructions, p 76
CONTINUING CARE: p 78
PREVENTION: p 79

FOOT STRAIN: top

EXTENSOR TENDINITIS

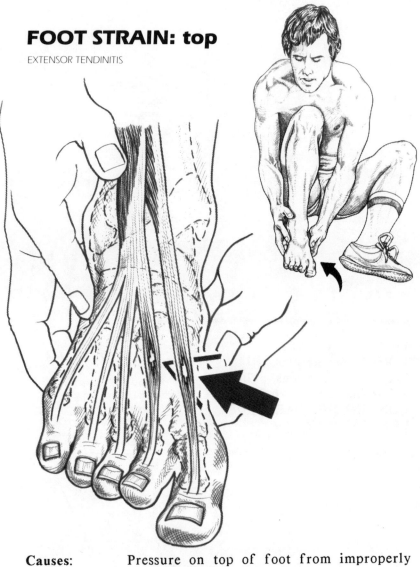

Causes:	Pressure on top of foot from improperly fitting athletic shoes or laces that are too tight. Made worse by running.
Effects:	Gradual irritation and strain of extensor tendon(s) on top of foot, causing mild to moderate tears.
Symptoms:	Inflammation and pain on top of usually only one foot.
Major Sports:	Any sport.
Healing Time:	About 1 week.

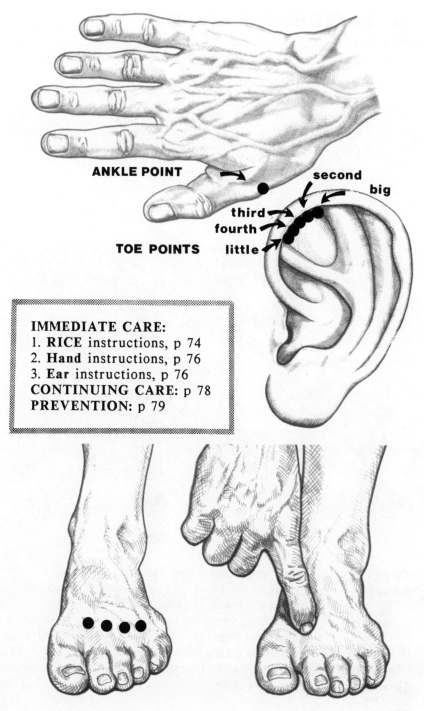

ANKLE POINT

second

big

third

fourth

TOE POINTS

little

IMMEDIATE CARE:
1. **RICE** instructions, p 74
2. **Hand** instructions, p 76
3. **Ear** instructions, p 76
CONTINUING CARE: p 78
PREVENTION: p 79

HAND STRAIN

FLEXOR TENDINITIS

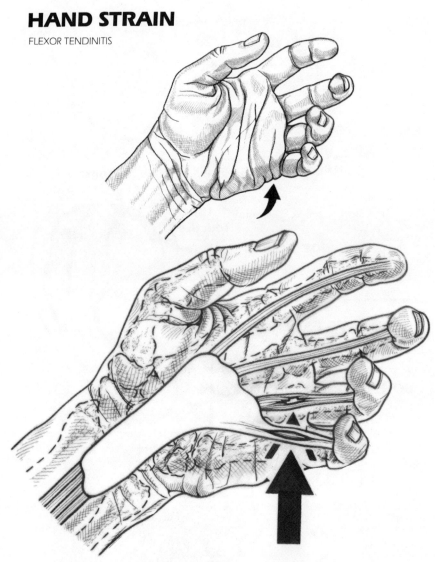

Causes: Overuse of hand and fingers.
Effects: Progressive (over 5 to 7 days) mild to moderate tears of lining of tendon tube.
Symptoms: Irritation, swelling of tendon tube, pain in palm and fingers, stiffness and difficulty in bending fingers into palm.
Major Sports: Baseball, Golf, Hockey and Tennis.
Healing Time: 1 to 2 weeks.

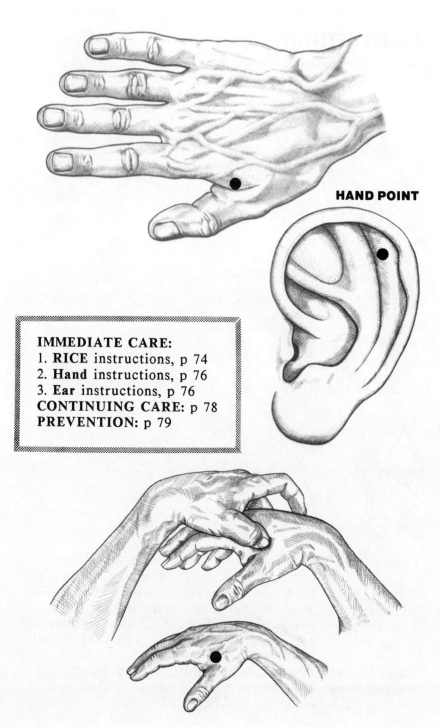

HAND POINT

IMMEDIATE CARE:
1. **RICE** instructions, p 74
2. **Hand** instructions, p 76
3. **Ear** instructions, p 76
CONTINUING CARE: p 78
PREVENTION: p 79

KNEE SPRAIN: deep

ANTERIOR CRUCIATE LIGAMENT SPRAIN

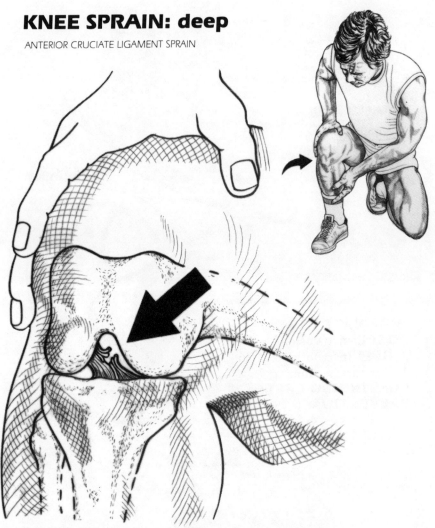

Causes:	External force applied to a bent knee or tremendous muscular force to knee.
Effects:	Mild or moderate tearing of middle ligament that connects the two leg bones.
Symptoms:	Tenderness, swelling and, sometimes, black and blue discoloration, with knee joint instability.
Major Sports:	Football, Lacrosse, Rugby and Soccer.
Healing Time:	Mild Sprain: about 1 week.
	Moderate Sprain: 2 to 3 weeks.

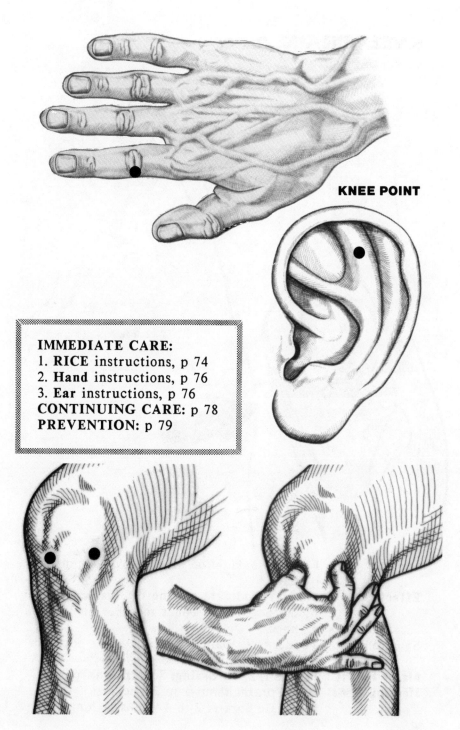

KNEE POINT

IMMEDIATE CARE:
1. **RICE** instructions, p 74
2. **Hand** instructions, p 76
3. **Ear** instructions, p 76
CONTINUING CARE: p 78
PREVENTION: p 79

103

KNEE SPRAIN: inner

MEDIAL COLLATERAL LIGAMENT SPRAIN

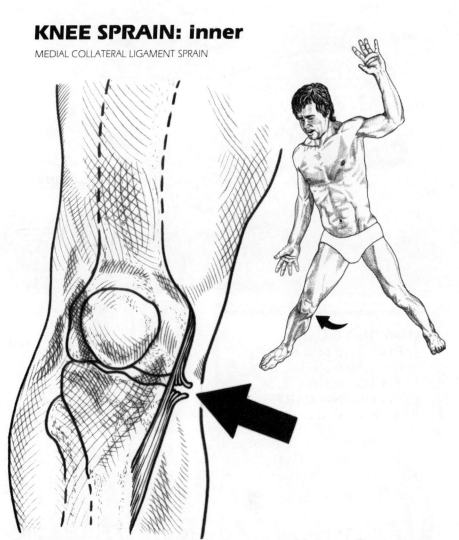

Causes:	Force to outside of knee or over-extension of knee.
Effects:	Mild to moderate tearing of ligament that holds the two leg bones together on inside of knee.
Symptoms:	Tenderness, pain, swelling and possible muscle spasm near knee.
Major Sports:	Football, Snow Skiing, Soccer and Tennis.
Healing Time:	Mild Sprain: about 1 to 2 weeks.
	Moderate Sprain: 2 to 4 weeks or longer.

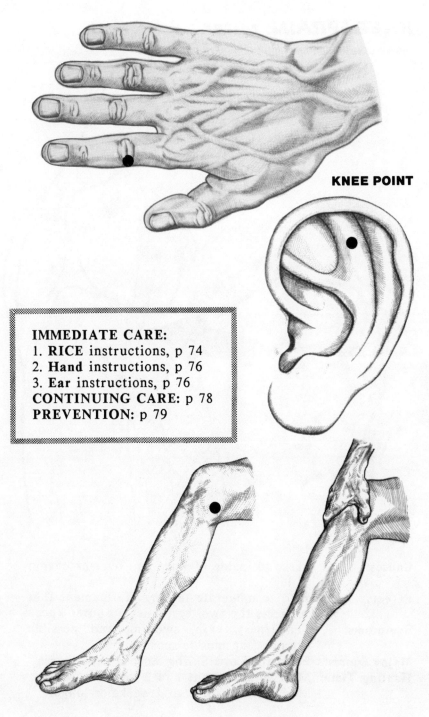

KNEE POINT

IMMEDIATE CARE:
1. **RICE** instructions, p 74
2. **Hand** instructions, p 76
3. **Ear** instructions, p 76
CONTINUING CARE: p 78
PREVENTION: p 79

KNEE SPRAIN: outer

LATERAL COLLATERAL LIGAMENT SPRAIN

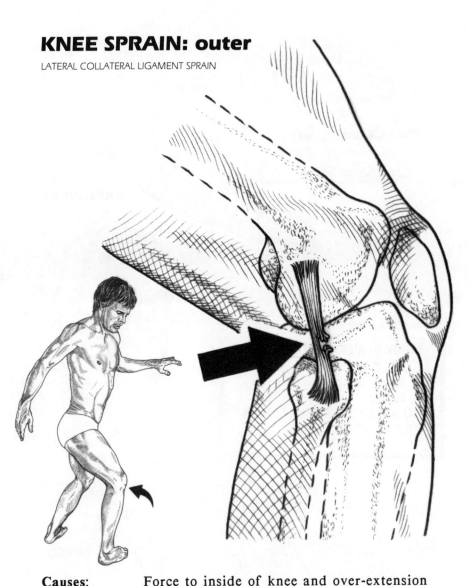

Causes:	Force to inside of knee and over-extension of leg.
Effects:	Mild to moderate tearing of ligament that connects the two legs bones on outer knee.
Symptoms:	Tenderness, pain, swelling and possible surrounding muscle spasm.
Major Sports:	Football, Snow Skiing, Soccer and Tennis.
Healing Time:	Mild Sprain: about 1 to 2 weeks. Moderate Sprain: 2 to 4 weeks or longer.

106

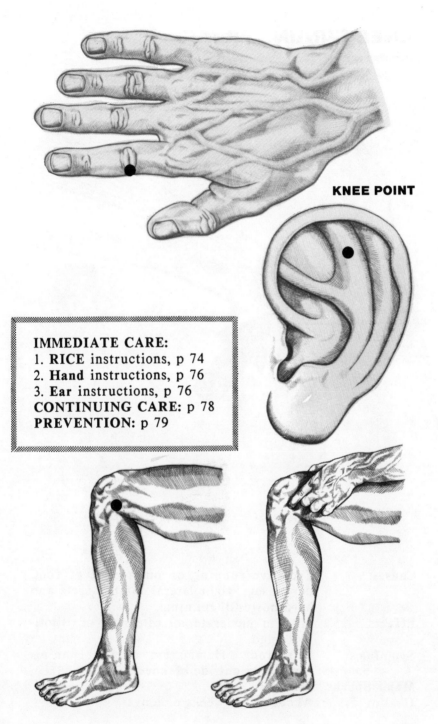

KNEE POINT

IMMEDIATE CARE:
1. **RICE** instructions, p 74
2. **Hand** instructions, p 76
3. **Ear** instructions, p 76
CONTINUING CARE: p 78
PREVENTION: p 79

KNEE STRAIN: outer

Runner's Knee

ILIOTIBIAL BAND TENDINITIS

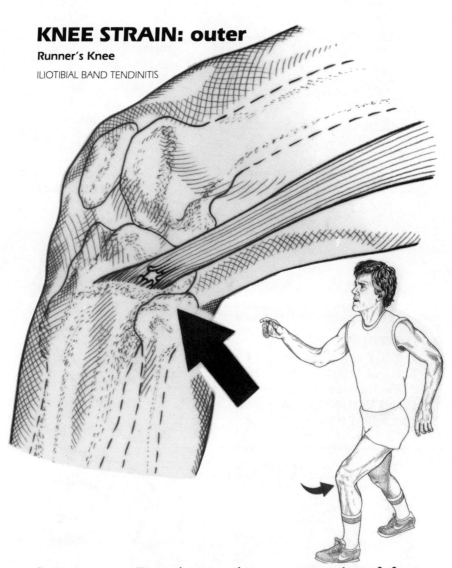

Causes:	Excessive running on outer edge of foot, bowed legs, tight lateral thigh muscle and hard downhill running.
Effects:	Mild to moderate microtearing of illiotibial band.
Symptoms:	Pain and inflammation during running, usually on outside of knee cap.
Major Sports:	Runners.
Healing Time:	About 4 to 6 weeks or longer.

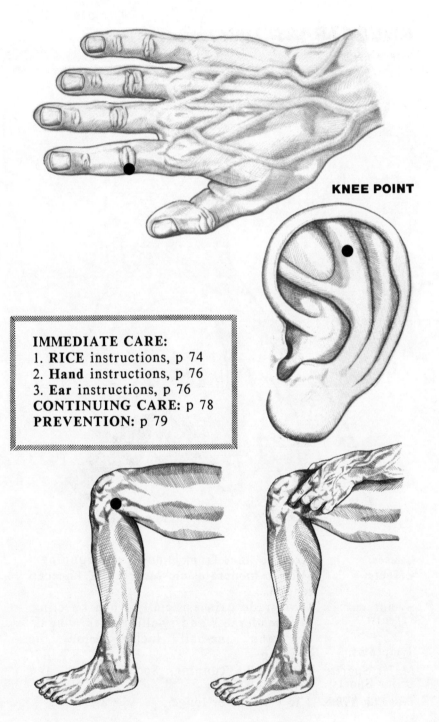

KNEE POINT

IMMEDIATE CARE:
1. **RICE** instructions, p 74
2. **Hand** instructions, p 76
3. **Ear** instructions, p 76
CONTINUING CARE: p 78
PREVENTION: p 79

KNEECAP STRAIN: lower

PATELLAR TENDINITIS

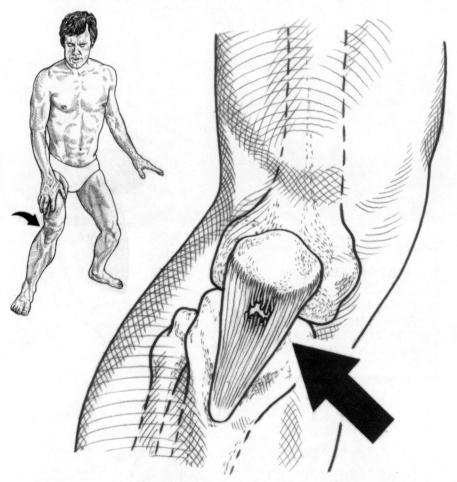

Causes:	Stress to knee from jumping and running.
Effects:	Mild to moderate microtearing of kneecap tendon.
Symptoms:	Low grade pain especially when kneeling; plus tenderness and swelling with a bump one and one-half inches below the kneecap.
Major Sports:	Basketball, Running, Soccer, Track and Volleyball.
Healing Time:	1 to 4 weeks or longer.

110

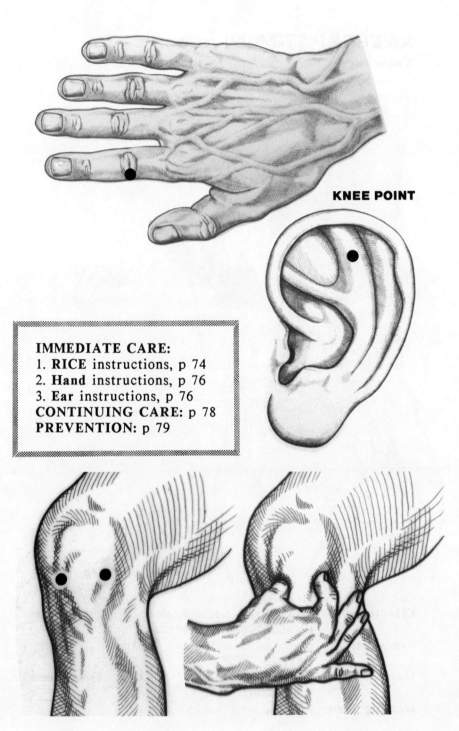

KNEE POINT

IMMEDIATE CARE:
1. RICE instructions, p 74
2. Hand instructions, p 76
3. Ear instructions, p 76
CONTINUING CARE: p 78
PREVENTION: p 79

KNEECAP STRAIN: upper

Jumper's Knee

QUADRICEPS TENDINITIS

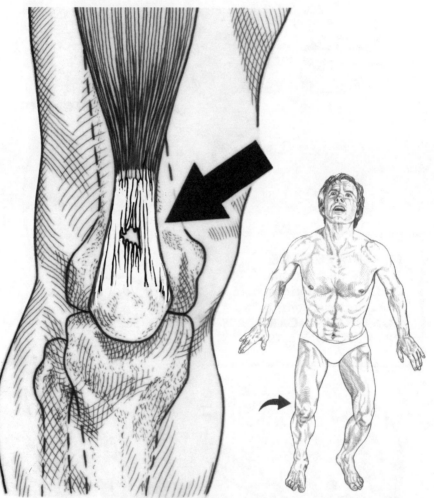

Causes:	Stress from jumping.
Effects:	Progressive microtrauma of tendon near its attachment to kneecap.
Symptoms:	Pain, especially when jumping or squatting, also tenderness and swelling.
Major Sports:	Basketball, Hurdlers, Long, High and Triple Jump and Volleyball.
Healing Time:	About 4 to 6 weeks or longer.

112

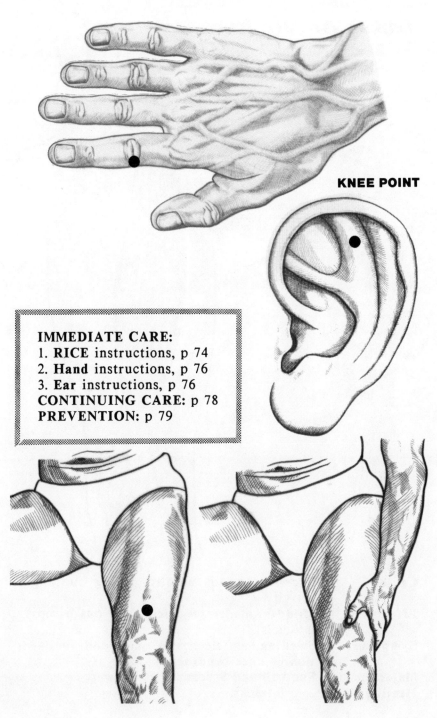

KNEE POINT

IMMEDIATE CARE:
1. **RICE** instructions, p 74
2. **Hand** instructions, p 76
3. **Ear** instructions, p 76
CONTINUING CARE: p 78
PREVENTION: p 79

THIGH STRAIN: front

QUADRICEPS MUSCLE STRAIN

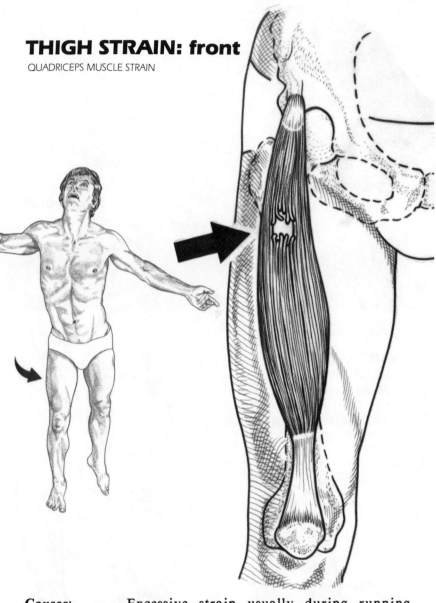

Causes:	Excessive strain usually during running activity.
Effects:	Mild to moderate tearing of quadriceps muscle(s).
Symptoms:	Swelling, muscle spasm, pain and limitation of knee bending.
Major Sports:	Football and Soccer.
Healing Time:	2 to 6 weeks.

114

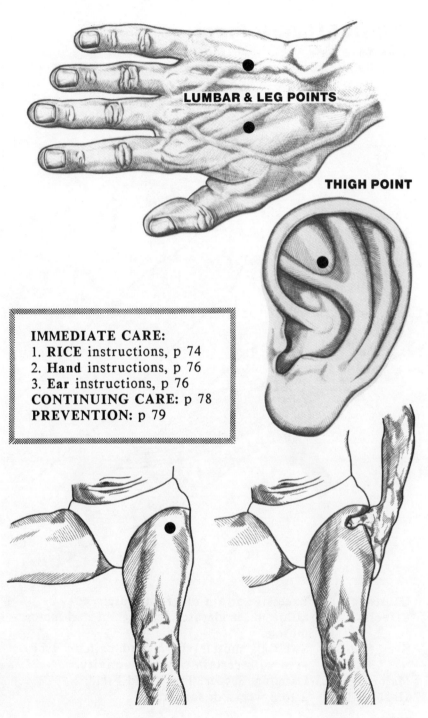

LUMBAR & LEG POINTS

THIGH POINT

IMMEDIATE CARE:
1. **RICE** instructions, p 74
2. **Hand** instructions, p 76
3. **Ear** instructions, p 76
CONTINUING CARE: p 78
PREVENTION: p 79

THIGH STRAIN: inner

Groin Pull

ADDUCTOR MUSCLE STRAIN

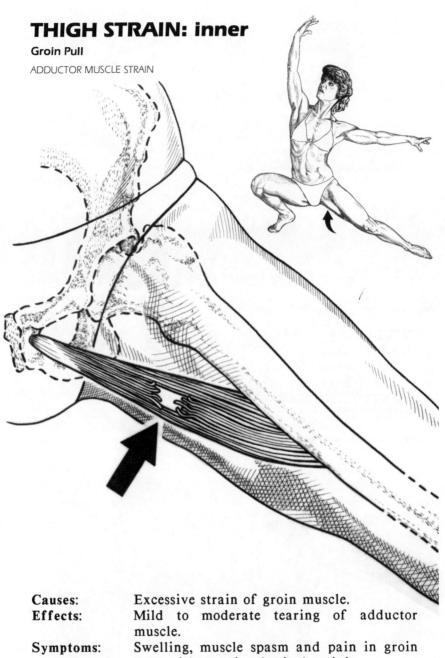

Causes:	Excessive strain of groin muscle.
Effects:	Mild to moderate tearing of adductor muscle.
Symptoms:	Swelling, muscle spasm and pain in groin area with certain physical activity.
Major Sports:	Dancing, Soccer, Track and Field.
Healing Time:	2 to 6 weeks or longer.

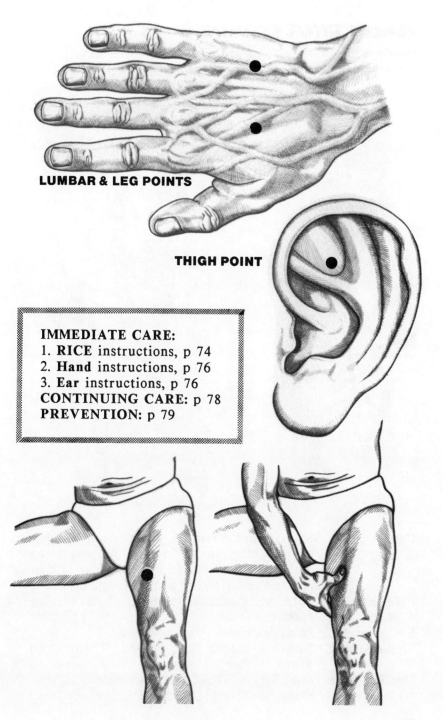

LUMBAR & LEG POINTS

THIGH POINT

IMMEDIATE CARE:
1. **RICE** instructions, p 74
2. **Hand** instructions, p 76
3. **Ear** instructions, p 76
CONTINUING CARE: p 78
PREVENTION: p 79

HAMSTRING STRAIN

HAMSTRING MUSCLE STRAIN

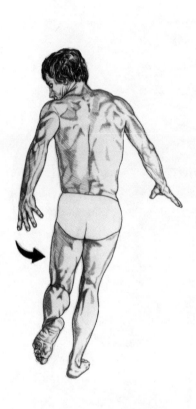 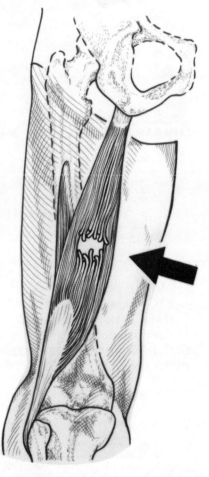

Causes:	Insufficient warm-up, extra strong quadriceps in relation to strength of hamstring muscle, lack of flexibility, stronger left or rigfht hamstring, or poor running style.
Effects:	Mild to moderate tearing of hamstring muscle.
Symptoms:	Pain, tenderness and swelling.
Major Sports:	Baseball, Basketball, Soccer, Tennis and Track.
Healing Time:	Mild Strain: about 1 to 2 weeks. Moderate Strain: 2 to 4 weeks.

118

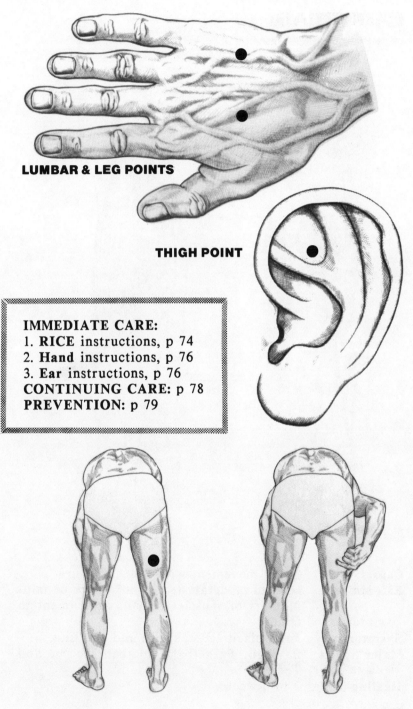

LUMBAR & LEG POINTS

THIGH POINT

IMMEDIATE CARE:
1. **RICE** instructions, p 74
2. **Hand** instructions, p 76
3. **Ear** instructions, p 76
CONTINUING CARE: p 78
PREVENTION: p 79

CALF STRAIN

GASTROCNEMIUS MUSCLE STRAIN

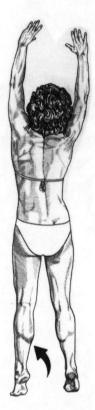

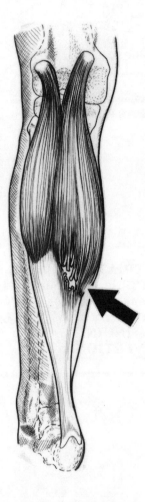

Causes:	Quick movement with foot tilted up.
Effects:	Mild to moderate tearing of upper or middle part of muscle from its attachment to tendon.
Symptoms:	Pain, often acute, spasm and swelling.
Major Sports:	Baseball, Basketball, Football, Soccer and Tennis.
Healing Time:	2 to 6 weeks.

120

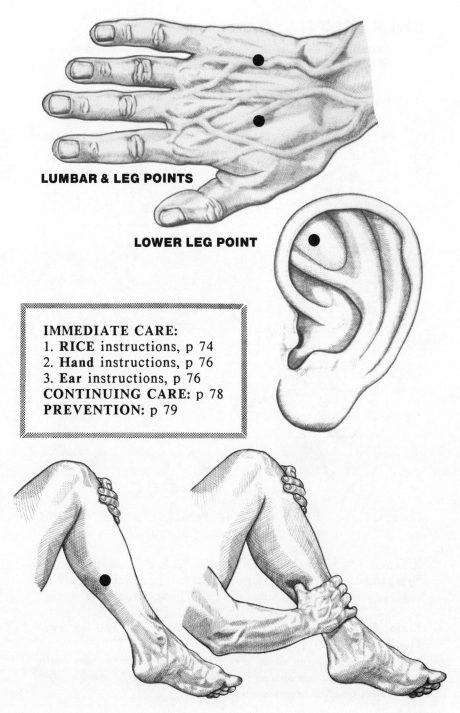

LUMBAR & LEG POINTS

LOWER LEG POINT

IMMEDIATE CARE:
1. **RICE** instructions, p 74
2. **Hand** instructions, p 76
3. **Ear** instructions, p 76
CONTINUING CARE: p 78
PREVENTION: p 79

SHIN SPLINTS: front

ANTERIOR TIBIAL,
EXTENSOR HALLUCIS AND/OR
EXTENSOR DIGITORUM LONGUS MUSCLE STRAIN

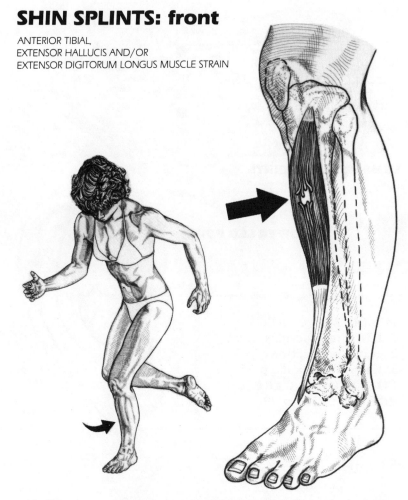

Causes: Excess running, which produces swelling and microtrauma in muscle covering of lower leg.

Effects: Lack of circulation to lower leg muscles.

Symptoms: Pain which is located parallel to and on outer side of shin bone area and which increases with running.

Major Sports: Basketball, Football, Running and Soccer.

Healing Time: 1 to 2 weeks.

NOTE: If you develop an intense lower leg pain that does not subside shortly after running, the condition may be **Acute Compartment Compression Syndrome.** Urgent medical help should be sought.

122

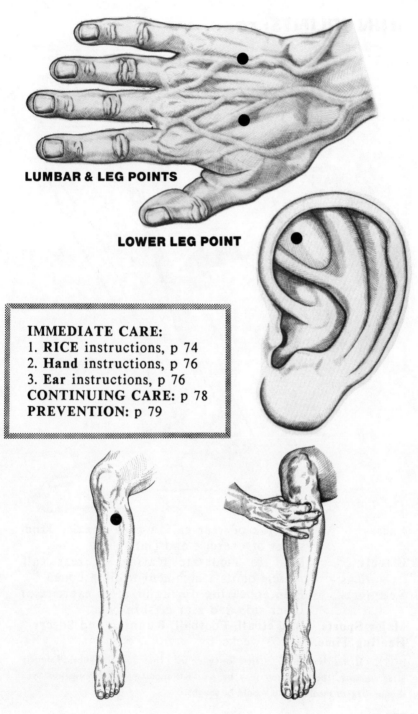

LUMBAR & LEG POINTS

LOWER LEG POINT

IMMEDIATE CARE:
1. **RICE** instructions, p 74
2. **Hand** instructions, p 76
3. **Ear** instructions, p 76
CONTINUING CARE: p 78
PREVENTION: p 79

123

SHIN SPLINTS: rear

POSTERIOR TIBIAL MUSCLE STRAIN

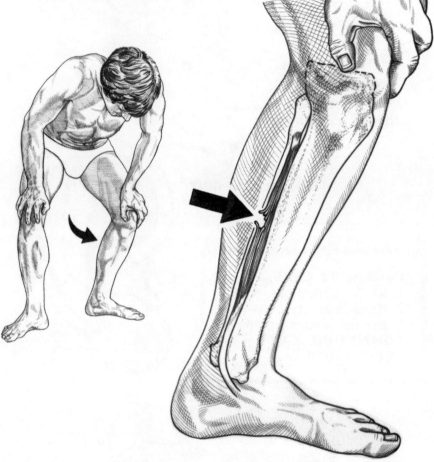

Causes:	Overuse of rear calf muscle usually from stress of exercise and flat feet.
Effects:	Mild to moderate tearing of rear calf muscle or its attachment to tibia bone.
Symptoms:	Pain appearing during or after exercise at inner side and rear of shin bone.
Major Sports:	Basketball, Football, Running and Soccer.
Healing Time:	2 to 3 weeks.

NOTE: If you develop an intense lower leg pain that does not subside shortly after running, the condition may be Acute Compartment Compression Syndrome. Urgent medical help should be sought.

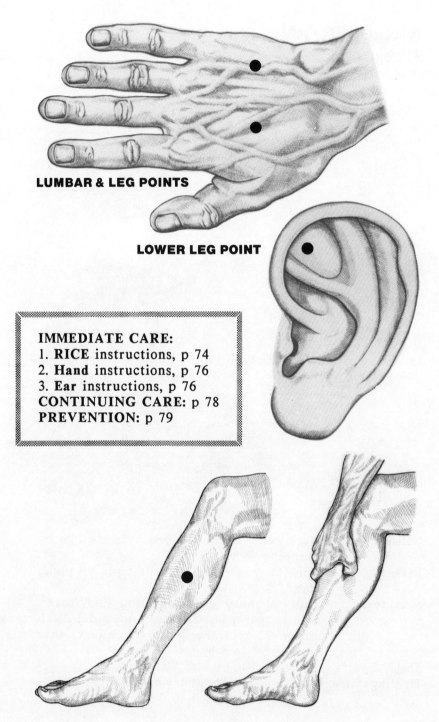

LUMBAR & LEG POINTS

LOWER LEG POINT

IMMEDIATE CARE:
1. **RICE** instructions, p 74
2. **Hand** instructions, p 76
3. **Ear** instructions, p 76
CONTINUING CARE: p 78
PREVENTION: p 79

NECK SPRAIN

Whiplash

CERVICAL SPINE LIGAMENT SPRAIN

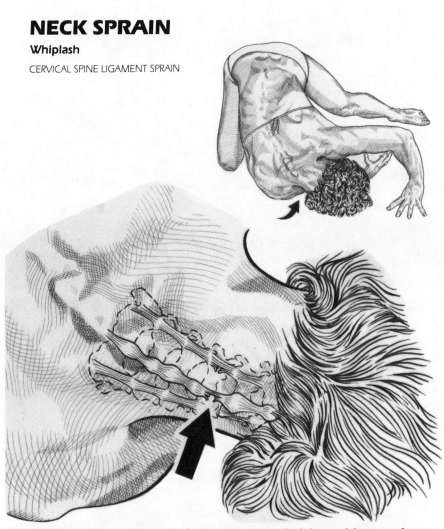

Causes:	Neck being over-extended by a blow or by snapping forward.
Effects:	Mild to moderate ligament tears of upper spine.
Symptoms:	Dull to sharp pain, swelling and, often, muscle spasm (usually only one side). Feels better 30 minutes following injury, then worse in 2 to 3 hours.
Major Sports:	Football, Rugby and Wrestling.
Healing Time:	Mild Sprains: about 1 week.
	Moderate Sprains: 1 to 2 weeks.

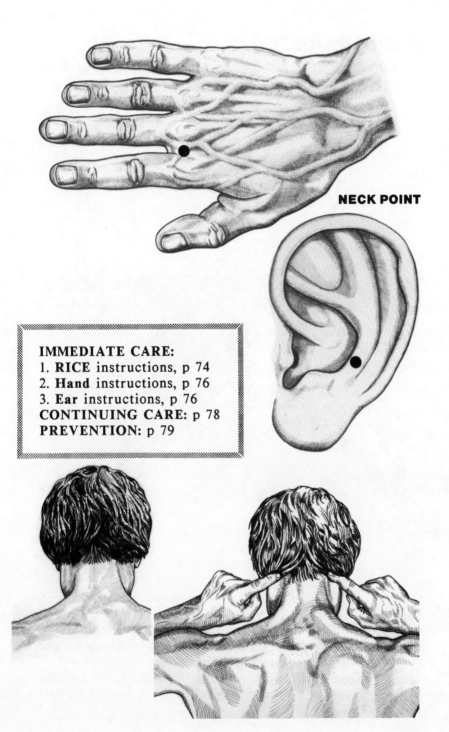

NECK POINT

IMMEDIATE CARE:
1. **RICE** instructions, p 74
2. **Hand** instructions, p 76
3. **Ear** instructions, p 76
CONTINUING CARE: p 78
PREVENTION: p 79

127

SHOULDER STRAIN

DELTOID MUSCLE STRAIN

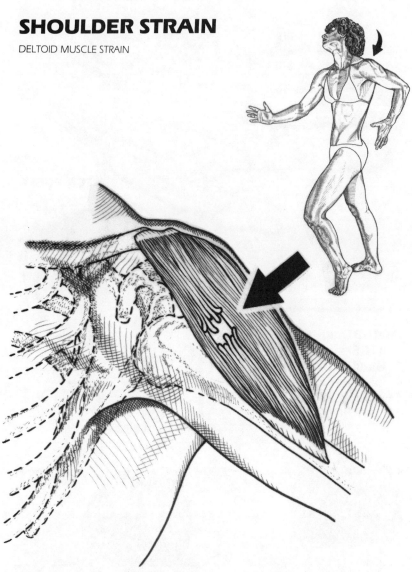

Causes: Overuse and over-extension.
Effects: Mild or moderate tearing usually at center of deltoid muscle.
Symptoms: Dull pain, swelling, spasm and discoloration of the skin.
Major Sports: Basketball, Football, Hockey, Lacrosse, Rugby and Soccer.
Healing Time: 2 to 4 weeks.

128

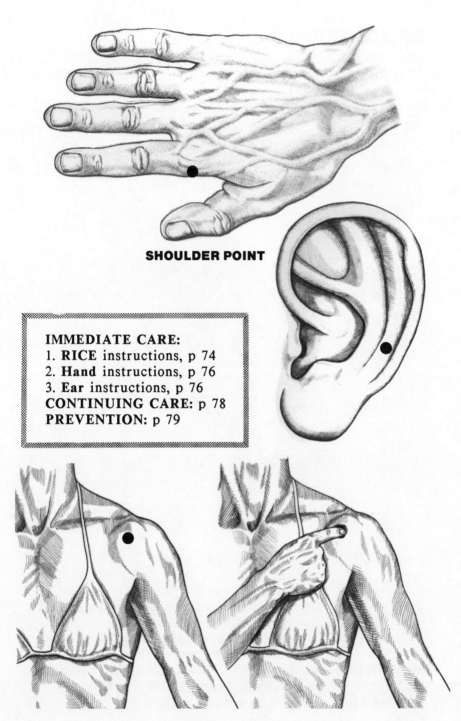

SHOULDER POINT

IMMEDIATE CARE:
1. **RICE** instructions, p 74
2. **Hand** instructions, p 76
3. **Ear** instructions, p 76
CONTINUING CARE: p 78
PREVENTION: p 79

BICEPS STRAIN

BICEPS TENDINITIS

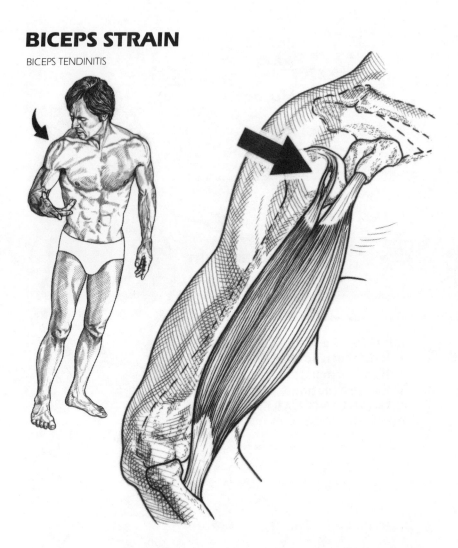

Causes:	Ligament injury which permits biceps tendon to slide in groove of upper arm or a deformity in arm bone groove.
Effects:	Mild to moderate microtears of tendon fibers at front of shoulder.
Symptoms:	Inflammation and pain at the site, especially when throwing or serving.
Major Sports:	Badminton, Baseball, Gymnastics, Racquetball, Tennis and Volleyball.
Healing Time:	About 4 to 6 weeks or longer.

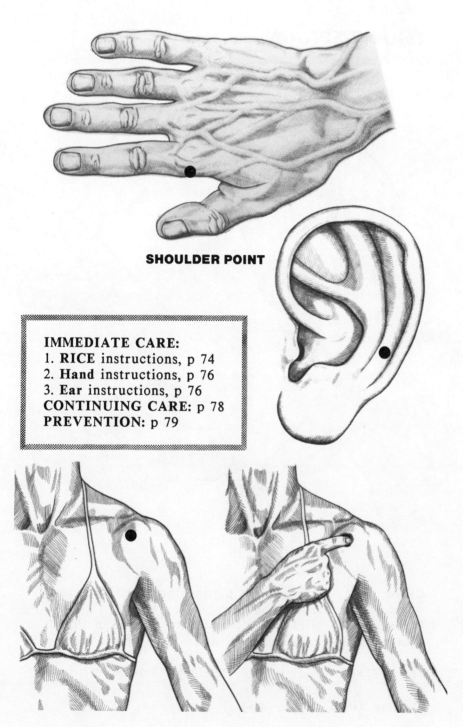

SHOULDER POINT

IMMEDIATE CARE:
1. RICE instructions, p 74
2. Hand instructions, p 76
3. Ear instructions, p 76
CONTINUING CARE: p 78
PREVENTION: p 79

THUMB SPRAIN

ULNAR COLLATERAL LIGAMENT SPRAIN

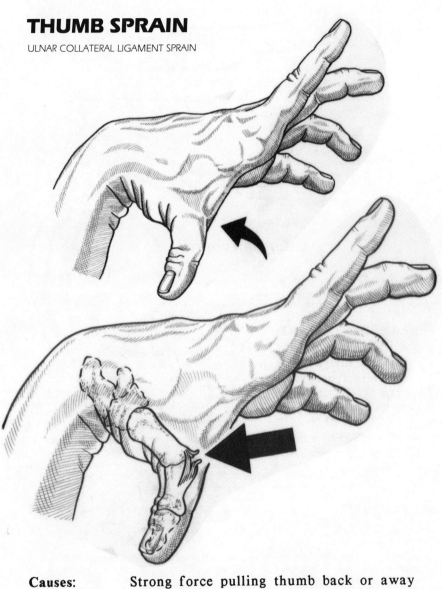

Causes:	Strong force pulling thumb back or away from hand.
Effects:	Mild to moderate ligament tears of thumb.
Symptoms:	Pain and swelling in weak area at base of thumb.
Major Sports:	Badminton, Baseball, Racquetball and Tennis.
Healing Time:	1 to 6 weeks.

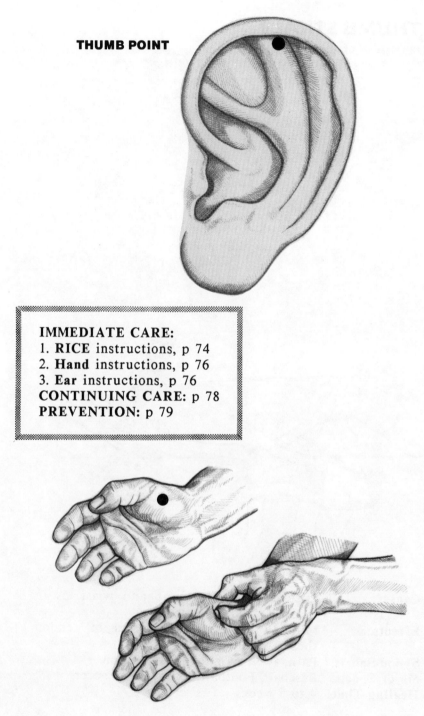

THUMB POINT

IMMEDIATE CARE:
1. **RICE** instructions, p 74
2. **Hand** instructions, p 76
3. **Ear** instructions, p 76
CONTINUING CARE: p 78
PREVENTION: p 79

THUMB STRAIN

DE QUERVAIN'S TENDINITIS

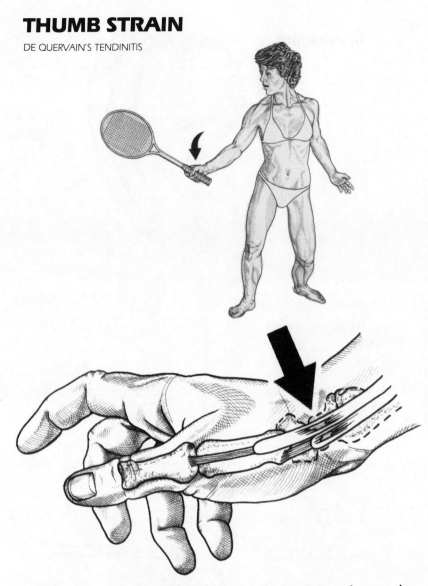

Causes:	Excessive use of thumb and wrist, as in throwing and racquet sports.
Effects:	Mild to moderate microtears of tendon sheath of thumb muscles.
Symptoms:	Pain, swelling and inflammation.
Major Sports:	Baseball, Football, Skiing and Soccer.
Healing Time:	4 to 6 weeks.

THUMB POINT

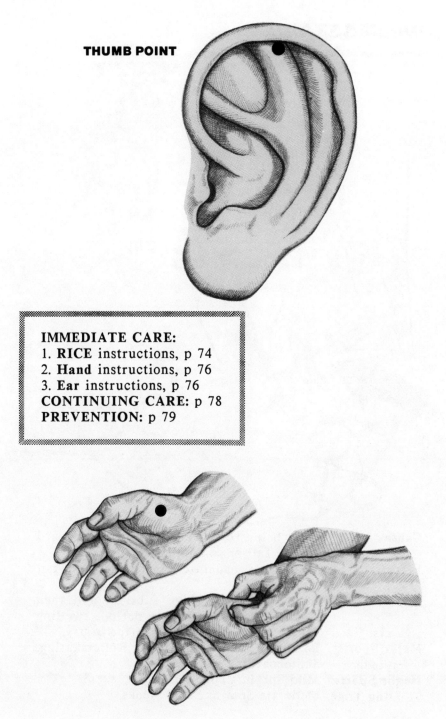

IMMEDIATE CARE:
1. **RICE** instructions, p 74
2. **Hand** instructions, p 76
3. **Ear** instructions, p 76
CONTINUING CARE: p 78
PREVENTION: p 79

WRIST SPRAIN

INFERIOR DORSAL RADIOULNAR LIGAMENT SPRAIN

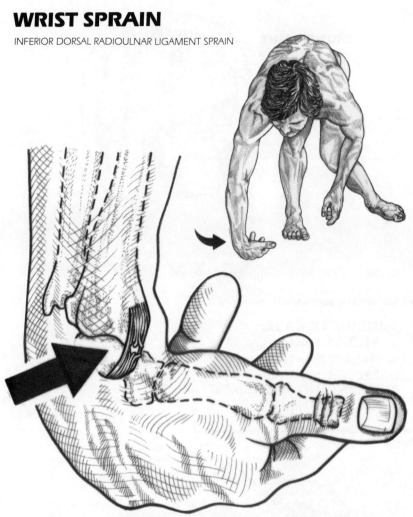

Causes:	Wrist being forced downward or backward as in a fall or contact sport.
Effects:	Mild to moderate tearing of wrist ligament.
Symptoms:	Immediate pain which subsides and then intensifies over a 3 hour period, swelling begins to appear one hour after injury.
Major Sports:	Boxing, Football, Hockey, Rollerskating, Skateboarding and Soccer.
Healing Time:	Mild Sprain: about 1 to 2 weeks.
	Moderate Sprain: 2 to 4 weeks.

136

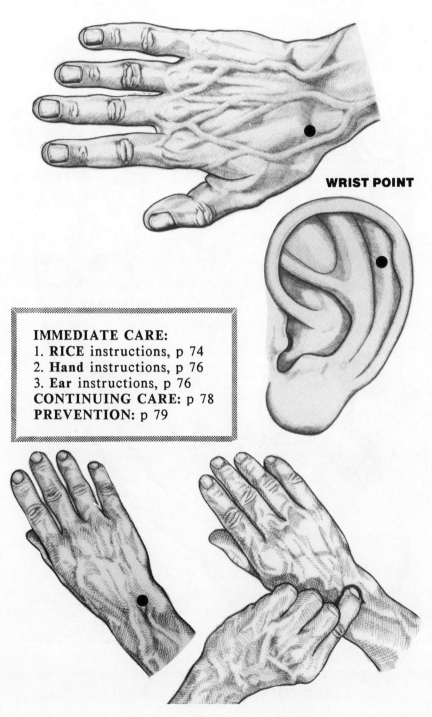

WRIST POINT

IMMEDIATE CARE:
1. **RICE** instructions, p 74
2. **Hand** instructions, p 76
3. **Ear** instructions, p 76
CONTINUING CARE: p 78
PREVENTION: p 79

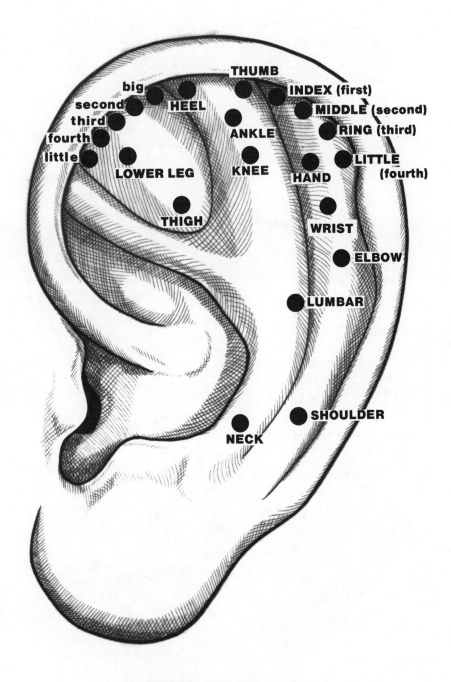

EAR POINTS CHART: treatment

138

History
of
Acupressure

The Chinese developed acupressure, which is merely the application of pressure to acupuncture points. Acupuncture itself involves stimulating the points with very fine needles, tapping, heat or electrical current. (Acu is derived from the Latin word *acus*, which means needle.)

Contrary to popular opinion, the use of acupuncture points, particularly on the ear, has not been limited to China. Doctors and scholars in India have stated that ear acupuncture was used there 2 to 3 thousand years before Christ and is still widely practiced today. Many countries have treatment systems similar to acupressure; the Japanese call their technique *Shiatzu*.

Along with the ancient cultures that use practices similar to acupuncture and acupressure, England and the United States are the sites of accounts from the early 1800's.

The first record of ear acupuncture in India is the *Suchi Veda, The Science of Needle Piercing*. Acupuncture in China has a documented history of over 2,000 years, but the records suggest it has been used there for almost 5,000 years. Although acupressure was probably used even before acupuncture, its first written account is a medical treatise from about 300 B.C. Found with the treatise were pencil-shaped stone needles with rounded ends, used for massaging and tapping certain body points.

Artwork from ancient Egypt shows a queen with a needle in her ear. It is not known whether Hippocrates, the father of Western medicine, was exposed to acupuncture while studying in Egypt, but he recommended ear stimulation for pain.

Sciatica, for instance, has been treated by the ear in many cultures for thousands of years. Ear treatment of sciatica has been effective when other methods fail. The Arabs used the ear not only to treat sciatica but also high blood pressure, kidney diseases and low back pain.

It wasn't until after World War II that a group of French physicians, led by Dr. Paul Nogier, began a careful study of the connections between the ear and various parts of the body. They were able to add many ear acupuncture points to those already in use. One of the discoveries that helped them map the exact ear acupuncture points was the realization that the ear resembles an upside down fetus.

Inspired by the French and their own curiosity, the Chinese launched a nationwide study of ear acupuncture. The French and Chinese efforts have located over 200 individual ear acupuncture points.

To find and confirm the best points for specific diseases or conditions, the Nanking Army ear acupuncture team conducted one of the largest medical studies in history during the late 60's and early 70's. These Chinese carefully analyzed the data from more than 200,000 treatments of over 20,000 patients. They obtained excellent results with 150 diseases.

They consistently found that stimulation of ear acupuncture points quickly and effectively kills pain, reduces inflammation, stops itching and reduces fever. It is used in emergency cases like shock, heat stroke and convulsions. These studies largely determined the development of modern ear acupressure.

Few studies have been done on hand acupressure, however the results are very satisfactory. Although scientific research on acupressure is small compared to that on acupuncture, those using both methods find that acupressure successfully treats many of the same conditions as acupuncture.

Over one-third of the world's population utilizes some form of acupuncture or acupressure. Why, then, has Western medicine only recently begun to seriously investigate the validity of these techniques? Because it functions from a philosophy of directly attacking the symptoms of disease through therapies that frequently require the use of drugs and/or surgery. In contrast, the Oriental philosophy behind acupressure strives for disease prev-

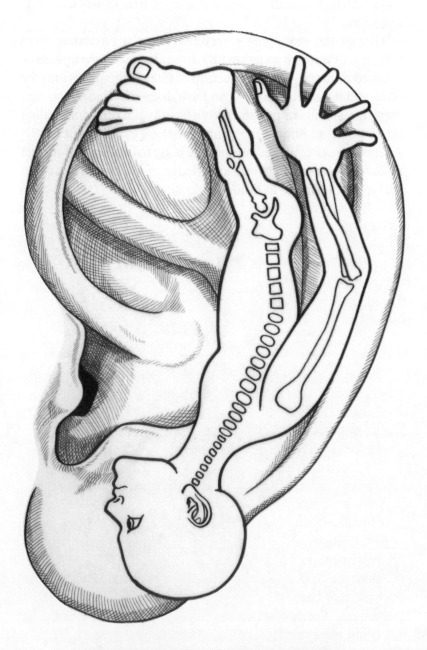

**Correlation of Ear Acupressure Points
and Human Musculo-Skeletal Structure**

ention through natural therapies that try to treat causes as well as symptoms.

Though the risks may sometimes make it advisable, most surgery cuts through some healthy tissue along with the injured or diseased portions. The introduction of foreign chemicals into the body and the use of surgery can have damaging side-effects that may permanently impair the body's healthy activities and healing processes. In addition, surgery and drugs are usually quite costly. Acupressure encourages and aids the body to balance and correct its own problems. Personal knowledge of acupressure can put health in your hands at little to no cost.

How
Acupressure
Works

There have been many theories proposed to explain the physiological function of acupressure. Some are now being accepted and
studied by Western Medicine. Further investigation of the connection between pressure points and the effected body parts will
create a more complete understanding.

The Chinese Meridian System

The oldest theory is the Chinese meridian system. Physicians in
ancient China discovered acupressure points through observation
that stimulation of specific points produces specific repeatable
responses even on remote parts of the body. Through painstaking
documentation of these findings, it was discovered that the points
are arranged in lines of similar effect. In other words, all the points
that effect a main organ, such as the stomach, seem to fall into a
definite line of energy flow along the body. These energy pathways are called meridians.

The Chinese concepts of meridians and acupressure are formed
around the balance of the dual yin/yang principles: the positive/-
negative, active/passive, male/female, complementary/opposite
aspects of the universe. Health is viewed as harmony of the whole
and illness as disharmony or lack of balance between the two
elements. To restore balance, certain acupressure points need only
be stimulated, which apparently balances by producing either a
stimulating or sedating effect.

Western medical science has been reluctant to accept the
meridian system as the basis of acupressure because it cannot be
directly related to a particular physical system within the body.

Some meridians follow the lymphatic or blood circulatory system to some extent; some may follow nerve pathways or sensory areas; and some seem to have no physical system counterpart. Some of the acupressure points are on or near nerves, but some are not related to major nerve locations at all; many but not all correspond to recognized trigger points. Of course, it is almost impossible to locate a point on the surface of the skin that is not near a sensory nerve.

Acupressure points can be electrically located and are viewed as part of the electromagnetic energy field of the body. The actual points lie just below the skin's surface. Though many different points may relate to a specific body function or part, some may be more therapeutically effective than others. Also, some single points may effect a wide variety of body functions or parts. Points lying along the same meridian have a complementary action, as do points on the corresponding left/right body sides.

The Nervous System and Acupressure

Some acupressurists believe that nerve pathways are the physical structure that facilitates acupressure. Nerve endings throughout the body are connected via the spinal chord to particular areas of the brain by a two-way system of nerve pathways. Thus, all parts of the body are interconnected. Hands and ears are richly supplied with sensitive nerve endings and thus are suitable sites for treatment of remote areas.

There are several theories as to the exact function of the nerves and the nervous system during acupressure. One theory that has found strong scientific support is that stimulation of certain acupressure points prompts the cerebral cortex, the hypothalamus and finally the pituitary gland to chemically release neurotransmitters and hormones, both inhibitory and excitatory. Endorphin and enkephalin, two hormones frequently associated with acupuncture, are morphine-like pain-inhibitors which can produce a *high* feeling. In addition, stimulation of the pituitary can further excite the adrenal glands to produce cortisone which can act as an anti-inflammatory agent.

144

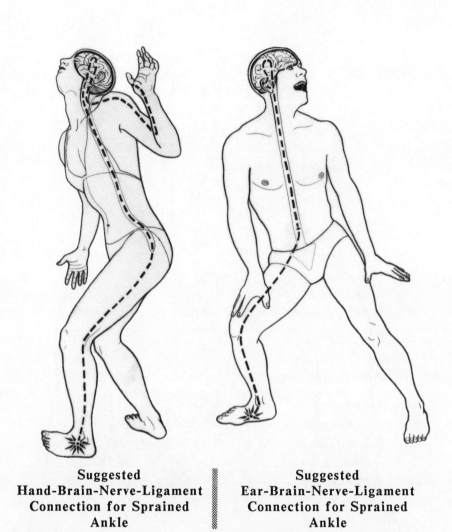

**Suggested
Hand-Brain-Nerve-Ligament
Connection for Sprained
Ankle**

**Suggested
Ear-Brain-Nerve-Ligament
Connection for Sprained
Ankle**

The Gate Control Theory

The gate control theory also involves the nervous system.
According to this theory, touch sensory stimulation sends pleasurable impulses to the brain, at a rate four times faster than painful
stimuli. The faster pleasurable impulses simply shut the neural
gates and the slower messages of pain never reach the brain. When
the brain does not receive painful stimuli, pain is not perceived in
the body.

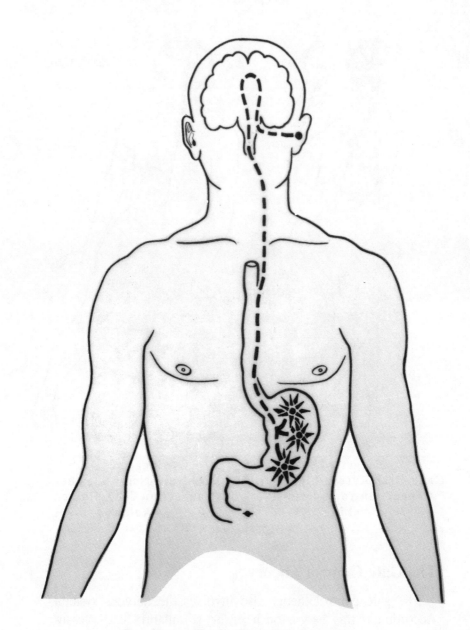

Ear-Nerve-Brain-Stomach Connection

The Circulatory System and Acupressure

A partial explanation of how acupressure alleviates pain in the body is put forth by those who feel that pain is merely the brain's perception that a cell or area of the body is experiencing too little or no oxygen: hypoxia or anoxia. Any circumstance that lessens circulation could cause hypoxia or anoxia because it is the blood that delivers oxygen to the cells. Traumatic injury could sever blood vessels. Over-use can create microtears and microtrauma that disturb or restrict blood flow. Even prolonged inactivity can cause circulation to become sluggish, and therefore cause muscles to ache. Since acupressure treatment improves blood circulation, more oxygen is available. This could then reduce or eliminate the perception of pain within the brain.

The Body's Electrical Energy and Acupressure

The bioelectric theory is based on physics rather than chemistry and states that stimulation of acupressure points alters the body's electrical potentials. Western medicine recognizes and utilizes changes in electrical potential through diagnostic machines such as the electroencephalograph (EEG), the electrocardiogram (EKG), and others less familiar. The effects of acupressure can be measured by an EEG and are usually toward a more relaxed state. This would indicate that rather than actually inhibiting the pain, acupressure lessens sensitivity to or perception of the pain.

That the body has an electromagnetic energy field or bioelectric energy field is, thus, scientifically accepted. The electromagnetic field has lines of force or energy flow which are invisible but which have measurable effects. Very simply, this could be compared to the lines of force that are visible when one puts iron filings on a magnet, because of the effect exerted on the filings. When the filings are removed, the lines of force are again invisible, though still present and still creating the electromagnetic field around the magnet.

The field itself is not of uniform intensity, but has areas of higher conductivity that coincide with the acupressure points.

Electroacupuncture equipment can measure the exact resistence of a given point. Every method of acupressure effects electrical balance at the point of stimulation and thereby effects the body's total electrical field and balance. Acupressure appropriately rectifies those points that are too low or too high, thus re-establishing balance. Imbalances seem to always precede sickness and are measurable before one is aware of any symptoms.

Every cell in the human body has an electrical potential and could be said to be polarized. Injury may have the effect of depolarizing those cells involved, thus creating an electrical imbalance in the involved area. Acupressure may enhance healing by reversing this depolarization and thus restoring the natural electrical energy flow within the body.

The interacting effects of acupressure include neural reactions, chemical reactions, electrical responses and changes, hormonal stimulation, and increased circulation of the blood and other body fluids. The one factor which could be called the common denominator of each of these reactions is the electric potential of every cell, which is an integral part of the body's over-all electrical field. Stimulation of the electric potentials can be brought about by chemical, electrical or mechanical means, as with acupressure. And the electrical responses themselves may then trigger neural, chemical and/or motor reactions. The bioelectric theory could lead to a scientifically sound explanation of acupressure identical in theory to the energy pathways inherent in the Chinese meridian system.

Acupressure Recommended Reading

BOOKS
For the Weekend Athlete

Finger Acupressure, Pedro Chan.
With over 525,000 copies sold, this is the most popular book on acupressure. It shows easy to find points for body pain and various health conditions.
New York: First Ballantine Books, 1975.

Ear Acupressure, Pedro Chan.
Another book by Chan; it follows a similar format as the one above, but for ear acupressure.
California: Chan's Corporation, 1977.

Acupuncture without Needles, J.V. Cerney.
This delightful book details the use of acupressure for ailments and pain. It shows many combinations of points.
New York: Cornerstone Library, 1974.

Shiatsu: Japanese Finger Pressure Therapy, Tokujiro Namikoshi.
Finger acupressure for sprains is briefly covered.
Tokyo: Japan Publications, Incorporated, 1972.

Sports Massage, Jack Meagher and Pat Boughton.
This book on massage includes acupressure points to treat injuries, thereby improving performance.
New York: Dolphin Books, Doubleday and Company, Incorporated, 1980.

The Sports Medicine Book, G. Mirkin and M. Hoffman.
The subject of sports medicine is covered in clear, easy style. Though not referred to by name, an acupressure technique is described as beneficial for stitches.
Boston: Little, Brown and Company, 1978.

BOOKS
For the Amateur to Professional Athlete

Touch for Health, John Thie.
This is the second most popular acupressure book: 225,000 have been sold. Use of neurolymphatic points for muscle pain and soreness are very helpful.
Marina del Rey, California: DeVorss and Company, 1979.

First Aid at Your Fingertips, Wood D. and J. Lawson.
This small, handy book tells how to use acupressure for pains, cramps and other sports ailments.
England: Health Science Press, 1963.

Chinese Massage Therapy, Anhui Medical School Hospital, China.
Sprains are covered in a nine page section, with case histories.
Translators Hor Ming Lee and Gregory Whincup. Boulder: Shambala, 1983.

The Sports Medicine Guide, Mark E. Wolpa.
This book deals specifically with common foot, leg and knee injuries and has numerous helpful photographs.
New York: Leisure Press, 1983.

Do-It-Yourself Shiatsu, Wataru Ohashi.
The reader is shown finger pressure on the body for relaxation and alleviation of painful conditions, and ear acupressure for weight control.
New York: E.P. Dutton, 1976.

Sports Health: The Complete Book of Athletic Injuries, William Southmayd and Marshall Hoffman.
This sports medicine book clearly illustrates and explains severe sprains and strains, however, there is no mention of acupressure or acupuncture and only one reference to effective use of trigger point therapy.
New York: Quick Fox, 1981.

BOOKS
For Coaches, Trainers and Health Care Professionals

Sports Medicine: Prevention, Evaluation, Management and Rehabilitation, Steve Roy and Richard Irvin.
This may be the best over-all book on sports medicine; it covers manual resistive muscle testing to determine muscular weakness and various massage techniques.
New Jersey: Prentice Hall, 1983.

150

Healing Massage Techniques: A Study of Eastern and Western Methods, Frances M. Tappan.
This excellent book combines massage and acupressure, describing benefits and physiological, body treatment points, plus the use of massage for athletes.
Reston, Virginia: Reston Publishing Company, Incorporated, 1980.

The Injured Athlete, Daniel N. Kulund.
Emphasis is placed on massage, trigger point therapy and acupressure for athletic rehabilitation and performance.
Philidelphia: J.B. Lippincott Company, 1982.

Sports Medicine: Fitness, Training, Injuries, Otto Appenzeller and Ruth Atkinson.
As *The Injured Athlete*, this book covers the use of massage, trigger point therapy and acupressure. A complete chapter on massage and sports is included. Both books have excellent bibliographies.
Baltimore: Urban and Schwarzenberg, 1983.

Muscle and Tendon Injuries in Athletes, Vladimir Krejci and Peter Koch.
This excellent medical book details when to use massage.
Stuttgart: Georg Thieme Publishers, 1979.

Tsubo: Vital Points for Oriental Therapy, Katsusuke Serizawa.
This well illustrated book on acupressure treatment points includes over 20 pages on treatment of muscles and joints.
Tokyo: Japan Publications, Incorporated, 1976.

Hit Medicine, Bob Flaws.
For those professionals more experienced with acupuncture and acupressure, this book is excellent. It describes injuries and prevention from the Oriental perspective. It also includes a great number of specific acupuncture points for injuries and improving sports performance.
Boulder: Blue Poppy Press, 1983.

MAGAZINE ARTICLES
For the Athlete

SPORTS FITNESS:

Pressure Point: Part I, David Nickel.
Part I includes the history of acupressure, how acupressure works and field studies with athletes.
July 1985, p 30-4 and 108.

Pressure Point: Part II, David Nickel.
Part II covers acupressure techniques plus how to treat athletic injuries and use acupressure points for warm-up, cool-down and pre-competition.
August 1985, p 28-32 and 94.

STRENGTH TRAINING:

Athletic Massage: Getting the Right Rub, Kim Goss.
This article shows you how massage and pressure point techniques can be used to alleviate soreness and improve performance.
October-November 1984, p 30-3.

NATIONAL STRENGTH AND CONDITIONING JOURNAL:

Massage for Athletes, Kim Goss.
An excellent article on the use of massage for restoring and toning injured muscle. Also includes the use of massage in competition.
January 1985, p 42c.

PHYSICIAN AND SPORTSMEDICINE:

The Neglected Art of Massage, Allan J. Ryan.
See the quotes from this Editor-in-Chief's editorial in the Introduction to this book, p 3.
December 1980, p 25.

Acupressure to Relieve Menstrual Cramps, B.E. Prentice.
Both the Effectiveness of acupressure for this condition and the technique for applying it are given in this article.
September 1981, p 171.

Trigger Point Massage Therapy, A. Peppard.
This article includes instructions on how to relieve upper body muscular tension.
May 1983, pp 159-62.

RUNNER'S WORLD:

Put Your Health in Your Hands, Don Monkerud.
Two of the first articles on acupressure in *Runner's World*, were by Don. This article will be of special interest to those that want to prevent injuries and enhance athletic performance. It discusses the use of acupressure by Dr. Leroy Perry for the most common running injuries: knee pain, shin splints and achilles tendinitis.
November 1976, pp 32-7.

Putting Your Finger on the Source of Pain, Don Monkerud.
This interview with the noted authority on acupuncture and acupressure, Dr. Ronald Lawrence, explains the use of acupressure on the skeleton to relieve pain and promote circulation and healing.
Volume 14, August 1979, pp 59-61.

Muscle Pulls and Cramps, Steven Roy.
The author suggests the use of massaging acupressure points to relieve cramps.
September 1983, p 37-9.

CHINA SPORTS:

Bone Setting the Traditional Way, Chen Geng.
Number 12, December 1983, p 20-1.

Massage Cures Insomnia, Diao Jinshan.
Number 9, December 1983, p 24.
Both of these articles advocate massage.

MAGAZINE ARTICLES
For Coaches, Trainers and Health Care Professionals

AMERICAN JOURNAL OF ACUPUNCTURE:

For the past 10 years, this publication has consistently offered top quality scientific articles on acupuncture.

A Comparison of Chinese and Nogier Auricular Points, T.D. Oleson and R.J. Kroening.
A helpful article for the effective choice of ear points.
Volume 11, Number 3, July - September 1983.

Acupressure as a Preventive Measure, as a Diagnostic Aid and a Treatment Modality, D.M. Beggs.
August 1980, pp 341-347.

PAIN:

Trigger Points and Acupuncture Points for Pain: Correlation and Implications, Ron Melzack, et al.
March 1977, pp 3-23.

POST GRADUATE MEDICAL JOURNAL:

The Myofascial Genesis of Pain, J. Travelle and S.H. Rinzler.
This article offers information important for an understanding of the use of acupressure and trigger points.
November 1952, pp 425-34.

SCINTIA SINICA:

The Role of Some Neurotransmitters of the Brian in Finger Acupressure Analgesia, Peking Medical College.
Volume 17, Number 1, February 1974, pp 112-30.

ADVANCES IN ACUPUNCTURE AND ACUPUNCTURE ANESTHESIA:

The Study on Finger Press Anesthesia, First Medical College of PLA.
This Chinese medical research paper records the findings of several studies on acupressure. It was used as the sole analgesia during extraction of upper and lower teeth on 3,488 patients, with a success rate of 97.8%. Tonsillectomy and maxillary sinus operations also using acupressure, had a success rate of 99.2% in 776 cases. In a comparison of acupressure and regular anesthesia for stomach operations, it was found that acupressure stabilized blood pressure more effectively and restored normal stomach function faster; 50% of the regular anesthesia group needed drugs to regulate their blood pressure.

Index

foot:
    pre-competition point 51
    sprain, arch 96
    strain, top 98
forearm, inner, flexor muscle strain 90
fracture healing 58
fright point, stage 47

G

gastrocnemius muscle strain 120
golf 29
good hurt, defined 10-11
Go-Power point 49, 51
groin pull 116
gymnastics 30

H

hamstring strain 118
handball 31
hand:
    acupressure technique 9, 76
    strain 100
    over-all warm-up point 21
headache relief 59
headaches 59, 64
heart burn 57
heat treatment 74
hoarseness 65
hockey, ice 32
hurt, good, defined 10-11

I

ice:
    as treatment 74
    hockey 32
iliotibial band tendinitis 108
indigestion 57
inflammation control 59
inner forearm flexor muscle strain 90
insomnia 58
intestine point, large 57
irregular menstruation 60
irritability 64
irritated joint 59
irritated muscles 59
irritated tendons 59

J

jet lag 61
joints, irritated and swollen 59
judo revival points 4
jumper's knee 112

K

kidney:
    injury 58
    point 58, 65
knee:
    jumper's 112
    runner's 108
    sprain, deep 102
    sprain, inner 104

sprain, outer 108
strain, outer 108
kneecap:
    strain, lower 110
    strain, upper 112

L

large intestine point 57
laryngitis 65
lateral collateral ligament sprain 106
lateral humeral epicondylitis 92
leg, over-all warm-up point 21
ligament:
    defined 69
    healing process 69-70
ligament sprain:
    anterior cruciate 102
    anterior talofibular 80
    cervical spine 126
    inferior dorsal radioulnar 136
    lateral collateral 106
    medial collateral elbow 88
    medial collateral knee 104
    proximal interphalangeal joint
        collateral 94
    ulnar collateral 132
Little League Pitcher's elbow 90
loss of appetite 56
lumbar strain 86
lung point 64, 65

M

martial arts 33
medial collateral ligament sprain:
    elbow 88
    knee 104
menstrual balance 60
menstruation, irregular and painful 60
microscars 71
microtrauma 71
microtears 71
mood elevation 60
motion balance 61
muscle:
    balance 61
    irritated and swollen 59
    relaxation 61
    relaxing point 47
    weakness 61
muscle strain:
    adductor 116
    anterior tibial 122
    calf 120
    defined 70-71
    deltoid 126
    extensor digitori m longus 122
    extensor hallucis longus 122
    forearm, inner, flexor 90
    gastrocnemius 120
    hamstring 118
    healing process 70-71
    posterior tibial 124
    quadratus lumborum 86
    quadriceps 114

156

Acupressure Personal Warm-Up and Cool-Down Form

NAME_____

SPORT_____

PURPOSE: Use the same acupressure points to stimulate your system before physical activity (warm-up) and to relax your system after your workout (cool-down).

ACUPRESSURE TECHNIQUE:

1. Apply continuous firm pressure to each appropriate point for 30 seconds: 5 seconds on - 5 seconds off. Begin on the right hand (or body side) and repeat to the left hand (or body side).
   - Move the corresponding (or opposite) body part as pressure is applied.
   - Visualize your body becoming stronger and more flexible, while exhaling forcefully.
2. Expect to feel:
   - Good hurt (an achy sensation) at each acupressure point.
   - Greater body strength and flexibility.

PART 1:

1. Circle and number the appropriate points to correspond with the hand warm-up diagram for your chosen sport. (Refer to Index for page number.)
2. Stimulate points 1, 2 and 3. Include more as an option.

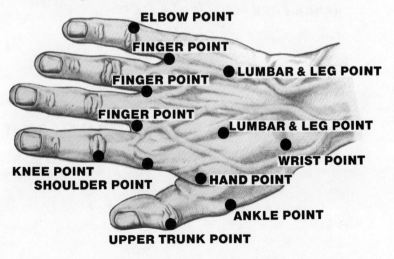

ELBOW POINT

FINGER POINT

FINGER POINT

LUMBAR & LEG POINT

FINGER POINT

LUMBAR & LEG POINT

KNEE POINT

SHOULDER POINT

WRIST POINT

HAND POINT

ANKLE POINT

UPPER TRUNK POINT

PART 2:

1. Circle the body point you are referred to in "Step 2" of your sport warm-up. Stimulate this point.
2. Optional: Circle the body points of previous injuries. (Refer to "Pain Chart" on page xiii.) Stimulate these points.

1_____ 2_____ 3_____

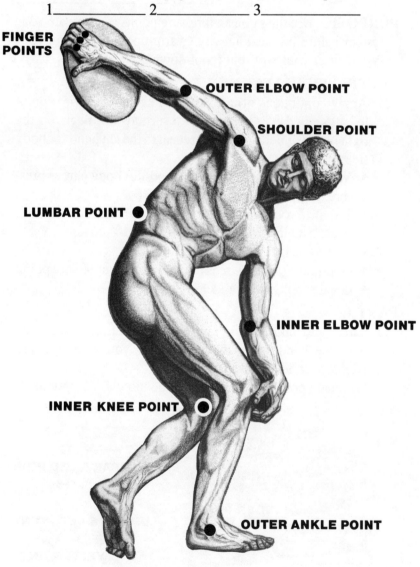

FINGER POINTS

OUTER ELBOW POINT

SHOULDER POINT

LUMBAR POINT

INNER ELBOW POINT

INNER KNEE POINT

OUTER ANKLE POINT

SPORTS FITNESS CHART

Acupressure does not supersede good medical service, but in emergency situations it can be used immediately while waiting for medical help. Also it can safely be used in conjunction with other treatments.

1. Allergies
2. Antiperspirant
3. Appetite Control
4. Bleeding
5. Breath relaxation
6. Common cold
7. Constipation
8. Coughing
9. Depression (Inside)
10. Diarrhea (use #7)
11. Dizziness
12. Drunk point
13. Eye pain
14. Fatigue (Inside)
15. Fever
16. Fracture
17. Headache in:
   F=front of head
   B=back of head
   S=side of head
   T=top of head
18. Hemorrhoids
19. High blood pressure
20. Indigestion
21. Inflammation (use #1)
22. Insomnia (Inside) (use #14)
23. Jet lag (motion sickness)
24. Muscle relaxant
25. Muscle spasm
26. Muscle weakness
27. Nasal congestion
28. Nervousness (stress)
29. Neurotic symptoms (use #23)
30. Pain: any type (use #28)
31. Painful menstruation (Inside)
32. Painful urination
33. Sciatica
34. Sexual Enhancement (Inside)
35. Shock (use #23)
36. Sore throat (Inside)
37. Steroid point (joint pain)
38. Testicular pain (Inside) (use #8)
39. Thirst point
40. Toothache

SUBSTANCE ABUSE
Alcohol
Cocaine
Caffeine
Marijuana   } (use Neurogate &
Tobacco   } Sympathetic points)
Tranquillizers
Antidepressants

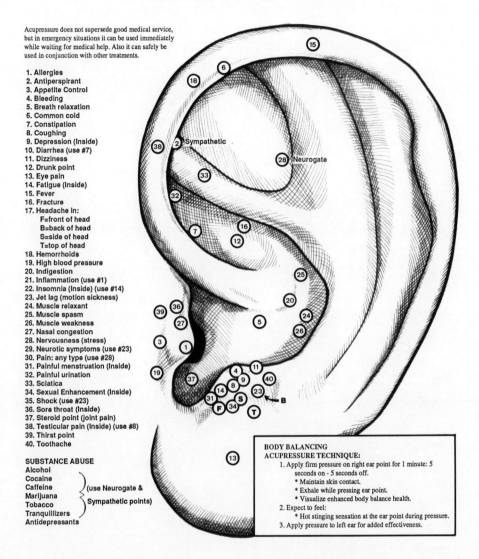

BODY BALANCING
ACUPRESSURE TECHNIQUE:
1. Apply firm pressure on right ear point for 1 minute: 5 seconds on - 5 seconds off.
   * Maintain skin contact.
   * Exhale while pressing ear point.
   * Visualize enhanced body balance health.
2. Expect to feel:
   * Hot stinging sensation at the ear point during pressure.
3. Apply pressure to left ear for added effectiveness.

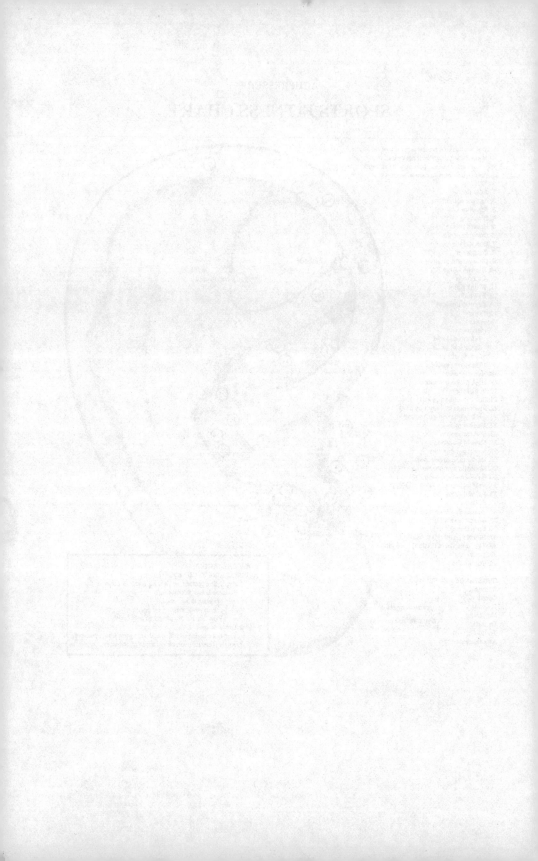